W9-CCI-615

Springer Series on the Teaching of Nursing

Diane O. McGivern, RN, PhD, FAAN, Series Editor
New York University

Advisory Board: Ellen Baer, PhD, RN, FAAN; Carla Mariano, EdD, RN, AHN-C, FAAIM; Janet A. Rodgers, PhD, RN, FAAN; Alice Adam Young, PhD, RN

Kathleen B. Gaberson, PhD, RN, CNOR, CNE, is Professor and Chair of the Department of Nursing Education and Director of Nursing at Shepherd University, Shepherdstown, West Virginia. She has more than 30 years of teaching experience in graduate and undergraduate nursing programs and has presented, written, and consulted extensively on teaching and evaluation in nursing education. Dr. Gaberson is Research Section Editor of the *AORN Journal*.

Marilyn H. Oermann, PhD, RN, FAAN, is a Professor in the College of Nursing, Wayne State University, Detroit, Michigan. She is author or coauthor of 11 nursing education books and many articles on clinical evaluation, teaching in nursing, and writing for publication. She is the Editor of the *Annual Review of Nursing Education* and *Journal of Nursing Care Quality*. Dr. Oermann lectures widely on teaching and evaluation in nursing.

Clinical Teaching
Strategies in Nursing
Second Edition

Kathleen B. Gaberson, PhD, RN, CNOR, CNE
Marilyn H. Oermann, PhD, RN, FAAN

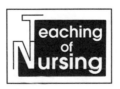

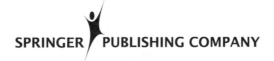

SPRINGER PUBLISHING COMPANY

New York

Springer Publishing Company, LLC
11 West 42nd Street
New York, NY 10036
www.springerpub.com

Acquisitions Editor: Sally J. Barhydt
Production Editor: Gail Farrar
Cover design: Joanne E. Honigman
Composition: Publishers' Design and Production Services, Inc.

09 10 / 5 4

Library of Congress Cataloging-in-Publication Data

Gaberson, Kathleen B.
    Clinical teaching strategies in nursing / Kathleen B. Gaberson, Marilyn H. Oermann. — 2nd ed.
      p ; cm. — (Springer series on the teaching of nursing)
    Includes bibliographical references and index.
    ISBN 0-8261-0248-4
    1. Nursing—Study and teaching.   I. Oermann, Marilyn H.   II. Title.
III. Series: Springer series on the teaching of nursing (Unnumbered)
    [DNLM: 1. Education, Nursing. 2. Teaching—methods.
WY.18 G112c 2006

RT73.G26 2006
610.73071—dc22

                                          2006051176

Printed in the United States of America by Bang Printing.

This book is dedicated to all teachers of nurse educators.

Contents

Contributors

Suzanne Hetzel Campbell, PhD, APRN-C, IBCLC
Assistant Professor
Fairfield University School of Nursing
Fairfield, Connecticut
Chapter 9, *Clinical Simulation*

Mickey Gillmor-Kahn, CNM, MN
Regional Clinical Coordinator
Frontier School of Midwifery and Family Nursing
Berea, Kentucky
Chapter 10, *Quality Clinical Education for Nursing Students at a Distance*

Susan E. Stone, DNSc, CNM, FACNM
President and Dean
Frontier School of Midwifery and Family Nursing
Berea, Kentucky
Chapter 10, *Quality Clinical Education for Nursing Students at a Distance*

Diane M. Wink, EdD, FNP, ARNP
Professor, School of Nursing
University of Central Florida
Orlando, Florida
Chapter 15, *Clinical Teaching in Diverse Settings*

Preface

Teaching in clinical settings presents nurse educators with challenges that are different from those encountered in the classroom. In nursing education, the classroom and clinical environments are linked because students must apply in clinical practice what they have learned in the classroom. However, clinical settings require different approaches to teaching. The clinical environment is complex and rapidly changing, and a transformed health care delivery system has produced a variety of new settings and roles in which nurses must be prepared to practice.

The second edition of *Clinical Teaching Strategies in Nursing* examines concepts of clinical teaching and provides a comprehensive framework for planning, guiding, and evaluating learning activities for undergraduate and graduate nursing students and health care providers in clinical settings. While the focus of the book is clinical teaching in nursing education, the content is applicable to teaching students in other health care fields in which students will interact with patients or clients. The book describes a range of effective and practical clinical teaching strategies that are useful for courses in which the teacher is on-site with students, in courses using preceptors and similar models, in simulation laboratories, and in distance education environments. It also examines innovative uses of nontraditional sites for clinical teaching.

The book begins with three chapters that provide a background for clinical teaching and guide the teacher's planning for clinical learning activities. Chapter 1 presents a philosophy of clinical teaching that provides a framework for planning, guiding, and evaluating clinical learning activities. This philosophy forms the basis for the authors' recommendations for effective clinical teaching strategies. Chapter 2 discusses the intended and unintended results of clinical teaching; it emphasizes the importance of cognitive, psychomotor, and affective outcomes that guide clinical teaching and evaluation. In Chapter 3, strategies for preparing faculty, staff, and students for clinical learning are discussed. This chapter includes suggestions for selecting clinical teaching settings and for orienting faculty and students to clinical agencies.

The next three chapters explore the process of clinical teaching. Chapter 4 discusses various clinical teaching models, including traditional, preceptor, and partnership forms. This chapter also addresses important qualities of clinical teachers as identified in research on clinical teaching effectiveness and the stressfulness of clinical teaching and learning. Chapter 5 describes the process of clinical teaching, including identifying learning outcomes, assessing learning needs, planning learning activities, guiding students, and evaluating performance. Chapter 6 addresses ethical and legal issues inherent in clinical teaching, including the use of a service setting for learning activities and the effects of academic dishonesty.

The next part of the book focuses on effective clinical teaching strategies. One of the most important responsibilities of clinical teachers is the selection of appropriate learning assignments. Chapter 7 discusses a variety of clinical learning assignments in addition to traditional patient care activities and suggests criteria for selecting appropriate assignments. This chapter includes new content on service-learning activities. Chapter 8 focuses on self-directed learning activities; it reviews various approaches to meeting the individual needs of learners through the use of multimedia and computer-assisted instruction as well as more traditional print resources. In Chapter 9, the use of clinical simulation to supplement actual clinical learning activities is discussed, including suggestions for designing simulation scenarios and running them effectively. Chapter 10 describes one graduate nursing program's approach to clinical teaching in a distance learning program. The suggested strategies are applicable to a wide variety of graduate and undergraduate nursing education programs. Chapter 11 discusses the use of case method, case study, and grand rounds as clinical teaching strategies to guide the development of problem solving, decision making, and critical thinking skills. In Chapter 12, the role of conferences and discussions in clinical learning is explored. Effective ways to plan and conduct clinical conferences, questioning to encourage exchange of ideas and higher-level thinking, and the roles of the teacher and learners in discussions and conferences are presented.

Chapter 13 focuses on written assignments of various types, including short written assignments for critical thinking, journals, concept maps, and portfolios, among others. Suggestions are made for selecting and evaluating a variety of assignments related to important clinical outcomes. Chapter 14 describes effective strategies for using preceptors in clinical teaching. The selection, preparation, and evaluation of preceptors are discussed, and the advantages and disadvantages of using preceptors are explored. This chapter also discusses the use of learning contracts as a strategy for planning and implementing preceptorships. Chapter 15 presents examples of effective ways to use diverse settings such as community-based, international, and underused traditional patient care sites for clinical learning activities.

Chapter 16, the final chapter, is new to this edition and focuses on the critical issue of clinical evaluation and grading. It is a succinct summary of three chapters in the authors' text, *Evaluation and Testing in Nursing Education*, 2nd edition (Oermann & Gaberson, 2006, Springer Publishing Company), and readers are referred to this companion book for a more extensive discussion of that topic. With the addition of this new chapter, *Clinical Teaching Strategies in Nursing* is a comprehensive source of information for full-time and part-time faculty members whose responsibilities largely center on clinical teaching.

Our thinking about and practice of clinical teaching has been shaped over many years by a number of teachers, mentors, and colleagues as well as through our own clinical teaching experience. It is impossible to acknowledge the specific contributions of each, but we hope that by the publication of this book they will know how much they have influenced us as teachers. Although we now cannot identify the sources of many ideas that we have gradually formed into our own framework for clinical teaching, we wish to acknowledge the origin of two ideas discussed in this book. The concept of essential and enrichment curricula came from G. Bradley Seager, Jr. The notion that every clinical teacher has a philosophy of clinical teaching, whether or not the teacher knows it, was adapted from Elizabeth Whalen's philosophy of editing, whether or not she knows it.

We thank Sally Barhydt for her patience and encouragement.

Kathleen B. Gaberson
Marilyn H. Oermann

Chapter 1

A Philosophy of Clinical Teaching

Every clinical teacher has a philosophy of clinical teaching, whether or not the teacher realizes it. That philosophy determines the teacher's understanding of his or her role, approaches to clinical teaching, selection of teaching and learning activities, use of evaluation processes, and relationships with learners and others in the clinical environment.

This book provides a framework for planning, guiding, and evaluating the clinical learning activities of nursing students and health care providers based on the authors' philosophy of clinical teaching. That philosophy of clinical teaching is discussed in this chapter. Readers may not agree with every element of the philosophy, but they should be able to see congruence between what the authors believe about clinical teaching and the recommendations they make to guide effective clinical teaching. Readers are encouraged to articulate their personal philosophies of nursing education in general and clinical teaching in particular to guide their own clinical teaching practice.

WHAT IS A PHILOSOPHY OF CLINICAL TEACHING?

In the sense that it is used most frequently in education, a *philosophy* is a system of shared beliefs and values held by members of an academic or practice discipline. Philosophy as a comprehensive scientific discipline focuses on more than beliefs, but beliefs determine the direction of science and thus form a basis for examining knowledge in any science. In the modern sciences, it is taken for granted that every scientist has and needs a philosophy (Uys & Smit, 1994).

Philosophical statements serve as a guide for examining issues and determining the priorities of a discipline (Butcher, 2004; Iwasiw, Goldenburg, & Andrusyszyn, 2005). Although a philosophy does not prescribe specific actions, it gives meaning and direction to practice, and it provides a basis for decision making and for determining whether one's behavior is consistent with one's beliefs. Without a philosophy to guide choices, a person is overly vulnerable to tradition, custom, and fad (Fitzpatrick, 2005; Tanner & Tanner, 2006).

An educational philosophy includes statements of belief about the goals of education, the nature of teaching and learning, and the roles of learners and teachers (Iwasiw et al., 2005). It provides a framework for making curricular and instructional choices and decisions from among options. The values and beliefs included in an educational philosophy provide structure and coherence for a curriculum, but statements of philosophy are meaningless if they are contradicted by actual educational practice (Dillard, Sitkberg, & Laidig, 2005; Tanner & Tanner, 2006). In nursing education, a philosophy directs the curriculum development process by providing a basis for selecting, sequencing, and using content and learning activities (Iwasiw et al., 2005).

The development and periodic examination of a shared philosophy of nursing education can guide professional development and lay the foundation for a common sense of identity among the faculty (Iwasiw et al., 2005; Uys & Smit, 1994). Each individual nurse educator has an educational philosophy that contextualizes, frames, and focuses his or her teaching activity, whether or not the nurse educator is aware of it (O'Mara, Carpio, Mallette, Down, & Brown, 2000; Petress, 2003). An educational philosophy comprises the "assumptions, goals, choices, attitudes, and values" that determine how the educator perceives the task of teaching and the means by which he or she carries it out (Iwasiw et al., 2005, p. 128).

In nursing and other health care professions, one important type of educational philosophy is a philosophy of *clinical* teaching, a set of beliefs about the purposes of clinical education and the responsibilities of teachers and learners in clinical settings. To become more effective clinical teachers, nurse educators first must reflect on their fundamental beliefs and assumptions about the value of clinical education, the roles and relationships of teachers and learners, and how desired outcomes are best achieved. These beliefs serve as a guide to action, and they profoundly affect how clinical teachers practice, how students learn, and how learning outcomes are evaluated. Reflecting on the philosophical basis for one's clinical teaching can evoke anxiety about exposing oneself and one's practice to scrutiny, but this self-reflection is a meaningful basis for continued professional development as a nurse educator (O'Mara, et al., 2000).

A LEXICON OF CLINICAL TEACHING

Language has power to shape thinking, and the choice and use of words can affect the way a teacher thinks about and performs the role of clinical teacher. The following terms are defined so that the authors and readers will share a common frame of reference for the essential concepts in the philosophy of clinical teaching.

Clinical

An adjective, the word *clinical* is derived from the noun "clinic," and it means involving direct observation of the patient. Like any good adjective, the word *clinical* must modify a noun. Nursing faculty members often are heard to say, "My students are in clinical today" or "I am not in clinical this week." Examples of correct use include "clinical practice," "clinical instruction," and "clinical evaluation."

Clinical Teaching or Clinical Instruction

The central activity of the teacher in the clinical setting is *clinical instruction* or *clinical teaching*. The teacher does not supervise students. Supervision implies administrative functions such as overseeing, directing, and managing the work of others. Supervision is a function that is more appropriate for professional practice situations than for the learning environment.

The appropriate role of the teacher in the clinical setting is competent guidance. The teacher guides, supports, stimulates, and facilitates learning. The teacher facilitates learning by designing appropriate activities in appropriate settings and allowing the student to experience that learning.

Clinical Experience

Learning is an active, personal process. The student is the one who experiences the learning. Teachers cannot provide a clinical experience; they can provide only the opportunity for the experience. The teacher's role is to plan and provide appropriate activities that will facilitate learning. However, each student will experience a clinical learning activity in a different way. For example, a teacher can provide a guided observation of a surgical procedure for a group of students. Although all students may be present in the operating room at the same time and all are observing the same procedure, each student will experience something slightly different. One of the reasons teachers require students to do written assignments or to participate in clinical conferences is to allow the teacher a glimpse of what students have derived from the learning activities.

ELEMENTS OF A PHILOSOPHY OF CLINICAL TEACHING

The philosophy of clinical teaching that provides the framework for this book includes beliefs about the nature of professional practice, the importance of clinical teaching, the role of the student as a learner, the need for learning time before evaluation, the climate for learning, the essential versus enrichment curricula, the espoused curriculum versus curriculum-in-use, and the importance of quality over quantity of clinical activities. Each of these elements of the philosophy is a guide to action for clinical teachers in nursing.

Clinical Education Should Reflect the Nature of Professional Practice

Nursing is a professional discipline. A *professional* is an individual who possesses expert knowledge and skill in a specific domain, acquired through formal education in institutions of higher learning and through experience, and who uses that knowledge and skill on behalf of society by serving specified clients. Professional disciplines are differentiated from academic disciplines by their practice component.

Clinical practice requires critical thinking and problem-solving abilities, specialized psychomotor and technological skills, and a professional value system. Practice in clinical settings exposes students to realities of professional practice that cannot be conveyed by a textbook or a simulation (Oermann & Gaberson, 2006). Schön (1987) represented professional practice as high, hard ground overlooking a swamp. On the high ground, practice problems can be solved by applying research-based theory and technique. The swampy lowland contains problems that are messy and confusing, that cannot easily be solved by technical skill. Nurses and nursing students must learn to solve both types of problems, but the problems that lie in the swampy lowlands tend to be those of greatest importance to society. Most professional practice situations are characterized by complexity, instability, uncertainty, uniqueness, and the presence of value conflicts. These are the problems that resist solution by the knowledge and skills of traditional expertise (Schön, 1983).

Because professional practice occurs within the context of society, it must respond to social and scientific demands and expectations. Therefore, the knowledge base and skill repertoire of a professional nurse cannot be static. Professional education must go beyond current knowledge and skills to prepare for practice in the future. Thus, clinical teaching must include skills such as identifying knowledge gaps, finding and utilizing new information, and initiating or managing change. Additionally, because health care professionals usually practice in interdisciplinary settings, nursing students must learn teamwork and collaboration skills (Oermann & Gaberson, 2006; Speziale & Jacobson, 2005).

Thus, if clinical learning activities are to prepare nursing students for professional practice, they should reflect the realities of that practice. Clinical education should allow students to encounter real practice problems in the swampy lowland. Rather than focus exclusively on teacher-defined, well-structured problems for which answers are easily found in theory and research, clinical educators should expose students to ill-structured problems for which there are insufficient or conflicting data or multiple solutions (Oermann & Gaberson, 2006).

Clinical Teaching Is More Important Than Classroom Teaching

Because nursing is a professional practice discipline, what nurses and nursing students do in clinical practice is more important than what they can demonstrate in a classroom. Clinical learning activities provide real-life experiences and opportunities for transfer of knowledge to practical situations (Oermann & Gaberson, 2006). Some learners who perform well in the classroom cannot apply their knowledge successfully in the clinical area.

If clinical instruction is so important, why does not all nursing education take place in the clinical area? Clinical teaching is the most expensive element of any nursing curriculum. Lower student-teacher ratios in clinical settings usually require a larger number of clinical teachers than classroom teachers. Students and teachers spend numerous hours in the clinical laboratory; those contact hours typically exceed the number of credit hours for which students pay tuition. Even if the tuition structure compensates for that intensive use of resources, clinical instruction remains an expensive enterprise. Therefore, classroom instruction is used to prepare students for their clinical activities. Students learn prerequisite knowledge in the classroom that they later apply and test in clinical practice.

The Nursing Student in the Clinical Setting Is a Learner, Not a Nurse

In preparation for professional practice, the clinical setting is the place where the student comes in contact with the patient or consumer for the purpose of testing theories and learning skills. In nursing education, clinical learning activities historically have been confused with caring for patients. In a classic study on the use of the clinical laboratory in nursing education, Infante (1985) observed that the typical activities of nursing students center on patient care. Learning is assumed to take place while caring. However, the central focus in clinical education should be on learning, not doing, as the student's role. Thus, the role of the student in nursing education should be primarily that of learner, not nurse. For this reason, the term *nursing student* rather than *student nurse* is preferred, because in the former term the noun *student* describes the role better than does its use as an adjective modifying the noun *nurse* in the latter term.

Sufficient Learning Time Should Be Provided Before Performance Is Evaluated

If students enter the clinical area to learn, then it follows that students need to engage in activities that promote learning and to practice the skills that they are learning before their performance is evaluated to determine a grade. Many nursing students perceive that the main role of the clinical teacher is to evaluate, and many nursing faculty members perceive that they spend more time on evaluation activities than on teaching activities. Nursing faculty members seem to expect students to perform skills competently the first time they attempt them, and they often keep detailed records of students' failures and shortcomings, which are later consulted when determining their grades.

However, skill acquisition is a complex process that involves making mistakes and learning how to correct and then prevent those mistakes. Because the clinical setting is a place where students can test theory as they apply it to practice, some of those tests will be more successful than others. Faculty members should expect students to make mistakes and not hold perfection as the standard. Therefore, faculty members should allow plentiful learning time with ample opportunity for feedback before evaluating student performance summatively.

Clinical Teaching Is Supported by a Climate of Mutual Trust and Respect

Another element of this philosophy of clinical teaching is the importance of creating and maintaining a climate of mutual trust and respect that supports learning and student growth. Faculty members must respect students as learners and trust their motivation and commitment to the profession they seek to enter. Students must respect the faculty's commitment to both nursing education and society and trust that faculty members will treat them with fairness and, to the extent that it is possible, not allow students to make mistakes that would harm patients.

The responsibilities for maintaining this climate of trust and respect are mutual, but teachers have the ultimate responsibility to establish these expectations in the nursing program. In most cases, students enter a nursing education program with 12 or more years of school experiences in which teachers may have been viewed as enemies, out to "get" students and eager to see them fail. Nurse educators need to state clearly, early, and often that they see nursing education as a shared enterprise, that they sincerely desire student success, and that they will be partners with students in achieving success. Before expecting students to trust them, teachers need to demonstrate their respect for students; faculty must first trust students and invite students to enter into a trusting relationship with the faculty. Setting up a climate of mutual trust and respect takes time and energy, and sometimes faculty will be disappointed when trust is betrayed. But in the long run, clinical teaching is more effective when it takes place in a climate of mutual trust and respect, so establishing such a climate is worth the time and effort.

Clinical Teaching and Learning Should Focus on Essential Knowledge, Skills, and Attitudes

Most nurse educators believe that each nursing education program has a single curriculum. In fact, every nursing curriculum can be separated into knowledge, skills, and attitudes that are deemed to be essential to safe, competent practice and those that would be nice to have, but are not critical. In other words, there is an *essential* curriculum and an *enrichment* curriculum. No nursing education program has the luxury of unlimited time for clinical teaching. Therefore, teaching and learning time is used to maximum advantage by focusing most of the time and effort on the most common practice problems that graduates and staff members are likely to face.

As health care and nursing knowledge grow, nursing curricula tend to change additively. That is, new content and skills are added to nursing curricula frequently, but faculty members are reluctant to delete anything. Neither students nor teachers are well served by this approach. Teachers may feel like they are drowning in content and unable to fit everything in; students resort to memorization and superficial, temporary learning, unable to discriminate between critical information and less important material. "Since it is impossible for faculty to teach everything that future nurses will encounter, nurse educators must be skillful in deciding what information is essential and how to teach it" (Speziale & Jacobson, 2005, p. 133).

Every nurse educator should be able to take a list of 10 clinical objectives and reduce it to 5 essential objectives by focusing on what is needed to produce safe, competent practitioners. To shorten the length of an orientation program for new staff members, the nurse educators in a hospital staff development department would first identify the knowledge, skills, and attitudes that were most essential for new employees in that environment to learn. If faculty members of a nursing education program wanted to design an accelerated program, they would have to decide what content to retain and what could be omitted without affecting the ability of their graduates to pass the licensure or certification examination and to practice safely. Making decisions like these is difficult, but what often is more difficult is getting a group of nurse educators to agree on the distinction between essential and enrichment content. Not surprisingly, in nursing education programs these decisions often are made according to the clinical specialty backgrounds of the faculty: The specialties that are represented by the largest number of faculty members usually are deemed to hold the most essential content.

This observation is not to suggest that the curriculum should consist solely of essential content. The enrichment curriculum is used to enhance learning, individualize activities, and motivate students. Students who meet essential clinical objectives quickly can select additional learning activities from the enrichment curriculum to satisfy needs for more depth and greater variety. Learners need to spend most of their time in the essential curriculum, but all students should have opportunities to participate in the enrichment curriculum as well.

The Espoused Curriculum May Not Be the Curriculum-In-Use

In a landmark guide to the reform of professional education, Argyris and Schön (1974) proposed that human behavior is guided by operational theories of action that operate at two levels. The first level, *espoused theory*, is what individuals say that they believe and do. Espoused theory is used to explain and justify action. The other level, *theory-in-use*, guides what individuals actually do in spontaneous behavior with others. Individuals usually are unable to describe their theories-in-use, but when they reflect on their behavior they often discover that it is incongruent with the espoused theory of action. Incongruity between espoused theory and theory-in-use can result in ineffective individual practice as well as discord within a faculty group.

Similarly, a nursing curriculum operates on two levels. The espoused curriculum is the one that is described on paper, in the self-study for accreditation or state approval and in course syllabi and clinical evaluation tools. This is the curriculum that is the subject of endless debate at faculty meetings. But the curriculum-in-use is what actually happens. A faculty can agree to include or exclude certain learning activities, goals, or evaluation methods in the curriculum, but when clinical teachers are in their own clinical settings, often they do what seems right to them at the time, in the context of changing circumstances and resources. In other words, every teacher interprets the espoused curriculum differently, in view of the specific clinical setting, the individual needs of students, or the teacher's skills and preferences. In reality, a faculty cannot prescribe to the last detail what teachers will teach (and when and how) and what learners will learn (and when and how) in clinical settings. Consequently, every student experiences the curriculum differently, hence the distinction between learning *activity* and learning *experience*.

When the notion of individualizing the curriculum is taken to extremes, an individual faculty member can become an "academic cowboy" (Saunders, 1999), ignoring the curriculum framework developed through consensus of the faculty in favor of his or her own "creative ideas and unconventional approaches to learning" (p. 30). Because a philosophy of nursing education is designed to provide clear direction to the faculty for making decisions about teaching and learning, the integrity of the program of study may be compromised if the practice of an individual clinical teacher diverges widely from the collective values, beliefs, and ideals of the faculty. Academic freedom is universally valued in the educational community, but it is not a license to disregard the educational philosophy adopted by the faculty as a curriculum framework. Thus, the exploration of incongruities between espoused curriculum and curriculum-in-use should engage the faculty as a whole on an ongoing basis, while allowing enough freedom for individual faculty members to operationalize the curriculum in their own clinical teaching settings.

Quality Is More Important Than Quantity

Infante (1985) wrote, "The amount of time that students should spend in the clinical laboratory has been the subject of much debate among nurse educators" (p. 43). Infante proposed that when teachers schedule a certain amount of time (e.g., 4 or 8 hours) for clinical learning activities, it will be insufficient for some students and unnecessarily long for others to acquire a particular skill. The length of time spent in clinical activities is no guarantee of the amount or quality of learning that results. Both the activity and the amount of time need to be individualized.

Most nursing faculty members worry far too much about how many hours students spend in the clinical setting and too little about the quality of the learning that is taking place. A 2-hour activity that results in critical skill learning is far more valuable than an 8-hour activity that merely promotes repetition of skills and habit learning. Nurse educators often worry that there is not enough time to teach everything that should be taught, but, as noted in the previous section, a rapidly increasing knowledge base assures that there will never be enough time. There is no better reason to identify the critical outcomes of clinical teaching and focus most of the available teaching time on guiding student learning to achieve those outcomes.

USING A PHILOSOPHY OF CLINICAL TEACHING TO IMPROVE CLINICAL EDUCATION

In the following chapters, the philosophy of clinical teaching articulated here is applied to discussions of the role of the clinical teacher and the process of clinical teaching. Differences in philosophy can profoundly affect how individuals enact the role of clinical teacher. Every decision about teaching strategy, setting, outcome, or role behavior is grounded in the teacher's philosophical perspective.

The core values inherent in an educator's philosophy of clinical teaching can serve as the basis for useful discussions with colleagues and testing of new teaching strategies. Reflection on one's philosophy of clinical teaching may uncover the source of incongruities between an individual's espoused theory of clinical teaching and the theory-in-use. When the outcomes of such reflection are shared with other clinical teachers, they provide a basis for curricular improvement and for the continual development of a sense of community within a faculty (Uys & Smit, 1994).

Nurse educators are encouraged to continue to develop their philosophies of clinical teaching by reflecting on how they view the goals of clinical education and how they carry out teaching activities to meet those goals. A philosophy of clinical education thus will serve as a guide to more effective practice and an effective means of ongoing professional development (Petress, 2003).

SUMMARY

A philosophy of clinical teaching influences one's understanding of the role of the clinical teacher and the process of teaching in clinical settings. This philosophy includes fundamental beliefs about the value of clinical education, roles and relationships of teachers and learners, and how to achieve desired outcomes. This philosophy of clinical teaching is operationalized in the remaining chapters of this book.

Terms related to clinical teaching were defined to serve as a common frame of reference. The adjective *clinical* means involving direct observation of the patient; its proper use is to modify nouns such as *laboratory, instruction, practice,* or *evaluation.* The teacher's central activity is *clinical instruction* or *clinical teaching,* rather than supervision, which implies administrative activities such as overseeing, directing, and managing the work of others. Because learning is an active, personal process, the student is the one who experiences the learning. Therefore, teachers cannot provide *clinical experience,* but they can offer opportunities and activities that will facilitate learning. Each student will experience a learning activity in a different way.

The philosophy advocated in this book contains the following beliefs: Clinical education should reflect the nature of professional practice. Practice in clinical settings exposes students to realities of professional practice that cannot be conveyed by a textbook or a simulation. Most professional practice situations are complex, unstable, and unique. Therefore, clinical learning activities should expose students to problems that cannot be solved easily with existing knowledge and technical skills.

Another element of the philosophy of clinical teaching concerns the importance of clinical teaching. Because nursing is a professional practice discipline, the clinical practice of nurses and nursing students is more important than what they can demonstrate in a classroom. Clinical education provides opportunities for real-life experiences and transfer of knowledge to practical situations.

In the clinical setting, nursing students come in contact with patients for the purpose of applying knowledge, testing theories, and learning skills. Although typical activities of nursing students center on patient care, learning does not necessarily take place during caregiving. The central activity of the student in clinical education should be learning, not doing.

Sufficient learning time should be provided before performance is evaluated. Students need to engage in learning activities and to practice skills before their performance is evaluated summatively. Skill acquisition is a complex process that involves making errors and learning how to correct and then prevent them. Teachers should allow plentiful learning time with ample opportunity for feedback before evaluating performance.

Another element of this philosophy of clinical teaching is the importance of a climate of mutual trust and respect that supports learning and student growth. Teachers and learners share the responsibility for maintaining this climate, but teachers ultimately are accountable for establishing expectations that faculty and students will be partners in achieving success.

Clinical teaching and learning should focus on essential knowledge, skills, and attitudes. Because every nursing education program has limited time for clinical teaching, this time is used to maximum advantage by focusing on the most common practice problems that learners are likely to face. Educators need to identify the knowledge, skills, and attitudes that are most essential for students to learn. Learners need to spend most of their time in this *essential curriculum.*

In clinical settings, the espoused curriculum may not be the curriculum-in-use. Although most faculty members would argue that there is one curriculum for a nursing education program, in reality the espoused curriculum is interpreted somewhat differently by each clinical teacher. Consequently, every student experiences this curriculum-in-use differently. A faculty cannot prescribe every detail of what teachers will teach and what learners will learn in clinical settings. Instead, it is usually more effective to specify broader outcomes and allow teachers and learners to meet them in a variety of ways. Individual faculty members are cautioned not to take individualizing the curriculum as a license to ignore the shared philosophy that guides curriculum development and implementation.

Finally, the distinction between quality and quantity of clinical learning is important. The quality of a learner's experience is more important than the amount of time spent in clinical activities. Both the activity and the amount of time should be individualized.

REFERENCES

Argyris, C., & Schön, D. A. (1974). *Theory in practice: Increasing professional effectiveness.* San Francisco: Jossey-Bass.

Dillard, N., Sitkberg, L., & Laidig, J. (2005). Curriculum development: An overview. In D. M. Billings & J. A. Halstead (Eds.), *Teaching in nursing: A guide for faculty* (2nd ed., pp. 89–102). St. Louis: Elsevier Saunders.

Fitzpatrick, J. J. (2005). Can we "escape fire" in nursing education? [Editorial]. *Nursing Education Perspectives, 26,* 205.

Haynes, L., Boese, T., & Butcher, H. (2004). *Nursing in contemporary society: Issues, trends, and transition to practice.* Upper Saddle River, NJ: Pearson Prentice Hall.

Infante, M. S. (1985). *The clinical laboratory in nursing education* (2nd ed.). New York: Wiley.

Iwasiw, C. L., Goldenberg, D., & Andrusyszyn, M, (2005). Developing philosophical approaches and formulating curriculum goals. In *Curriculum development in nursing education.* Boston: Jones and Bartlett.

Oermann, M. H., & Gaberson, K. B. (2006). *Evaluation and testing in nursing education* (2nd ed.). New York: Springer Publishing.

O'Mara, L., Carpio, B., Mallette, C., Down, W., & Brown, B. (2000). Developing a teaching portfolio in nursing education: A reflection. *Nurse Educator, 25,* 125–130.

Petress, K. (2003). An educational philosophy guides the pedagogical process. *College Student Journal, 37,* 128–134.

Saunders, R. B. (1999). Are you an academic cowboy? *Nursing Forum, 34,* 29–34.

Schön, D. A. (1983). *The reflective practitioner: How professionals think in action.* New York: Basic Books.

Schön, D. A. (1987). *Educating the reflective practitioner.* San Francisco: Jossey-Bass.

Speziale, H. J. S., & Jacobson, L. (2005). Trends in nurse education programs 1998–2008. *Nursing Education Perspectives, 26,* 230–235.

Tanner, D., & Tanner, L. (2006). *Curriculum development: Theory into practice* (4th ed.). Upper Saddle River, NJ: Pearson Prentice Hall.

Uys, L. R., & Smit, J. H. (1994). Writing a philosophy of nursing? *Journal of Advanced Nursing, 20,* 239–244.

Chapter 2

Outcomes of Clinical Teaching

To justify the enormous expenditure of resources on clinical education in nursing, teachers must have clear, realistic expectations of the outcomes of clinical learning. What knowledge, skills, and values can be learned only in clinical practice and not in the classroom?

Nurse educators traditionally have focused on the process of clinical teaching. Many hours of discussion in faculty meetings have been devoted to how and where clinical learning takes place, which clinical activities should be required, and how many hours should be spent in the clinical area. However, current accreditation criteria for higher education in general and nursing in particular focus on evidence that meaningful outcomes of learning have been produced. Therefore, the effectiveness of clinical teaching should be judged on the extent to which it produces desired learning outcomes.

This chapter discusses broad outcomes of nursing education programs that can be achieved through clinical teaching and learning. These outcomes must be operationally defined and stated as competencies and specific objectives to be useful in guiding teaching and evaluation. Competencies and specific objectives for clinical teaching are discussed in Chapter 5.

INTENDED OUTCOMES

Since the 1980s, accrediting bodies in higher education have placed greater emphasis on measuring the performance of students and graduates, holding faculty and institutions accountable for the outcomes of their educational efforts (Dillard, Sitkberg, & Laidig, 2005). Outcomes—the characteristics, qualities, or attributes that learners display at the end of an educational program—are the products of educational efforts. Teachers are responsible for specifying outcomes of nursing education programs that are congruent with the current and future needs of society. Changes in health care delivery systems, demographic trends, technological advances, and developments in higher education influence the competencies needed for professional nursing practice (Boland, 2005).

The historical approach to curriculum development as a process starts with a philosophy statement or a philosophical approach (Iwasiw, Goldenberg, & Andrusyszyn, 2005) and a conceptual, theoretical, or other curriculum framework that reflects this philosophy. Program goals are then developed, followed by more specific level and course objectives. Finally, content is selected and sequenced, and teaching strategies and evaluation methods are chosen to facilitate the attainment and assessment of the goals and objectives. This approach to curriculum design suggests a linear, mechanistic sequence of activities, which, in turn, implies that learning takes place in the same orderly fashion.

However, the curriculum reform movement of the 1980s focused on the importance of outcomes rather than process in improving the quality of teaching and learning in nursing education. This approach suggests that an orderly curriculum design does not take into account each learner's individual needs, abilities, and learning style, and that learners can reach the same goal by means of different paths. Development of the outcome-driven curriculum begins with specifying the desired ends and then selecting content and teaching strategies that will bring about those ends (Boland, 2005; Diekelmann, Ironside, & Gunn, 2005).

Thus, planning for clinical teaching should begin with identifying learning outcomes or competencies that are necessary for safe, competent nursing practice. These outcomes include knowledge, skills, and professional attitudes and values that are derived from the philosophical approach chosen to guide curriculum development.

Knowledge

Clinical learning activities enable students to transfer knowledge learned in the classroom to real-life situations. In clinical practice, theory is translated into practice. By observing and participating in clinical activities, students extend the knowledge that they acquired in the classroom and in self-directed learning. To use resources effectively and efficiently, clinical learning activities should focus on the development of knowledge that cannot be obtained in the classroom or other settings.

As discussed in Chapter 1, new content is added to nursing curricula frequently, reflecting the growth of new knowledge in nursing and health care. If the faculty is not willing to delete content that is no longer current or essential, the potential exists for creating a congested curriculum in which both students and teachers lose focus on the essential knowledge outcomes. Nurse educators thus need to develop evidence-based teaching skills that will help them to critically evaluate the evidence for content additions and deletions and decide what knowledge is essential for students to acquire (Speziale & Jacobson, 2005). For nursing education programs that prepare candidates for licensure or certification, consulting the licensure or certification examination test plans will help the faculty to focus attention on essential program content (Boswell & Cannon, 2005; National Council of State Boards of Nursing, 2004). The American Association of Colleges of Nursing publications, *The Essentials of Baccalaureate Education for Professional Nursing Practice* (1998) and *The Essentials of Master's Education for Advanced Practice Nursing* (1996) are helpful resources for selecting and organizing essential content in baccalaureate and graduate programs in nursing.

As an outcome of clinical teaching, knowledge encompasses both recall and comprehension of specific facts and information and knowing how to apply information to practice. Knowing how to practice nursing involves cognitive skill in problem solving, critical thinking, and decision making.

Problem Solving.   Clinical learning activities provide rich sources of realistic practice problems to be solved. Some problems are related to patients and their health needs; some arise from the clinical environment. As discussed in Chapter 1, most clinical problems tend to be complex, unique, and ambiguous. The ability to solve clinical problems is, therefore, an important outcome of clinical teaching and learning, and the nursing process itself is a problem-solving approach (Ignatavicius, 2004). Thus, most nurses and nursing students have some experience in problem solving, but complex problems of clinical practice often require new methods of reasoning and problem-solving strategies. Nursing students may not be functioning on a cognitive level that permits them to problem solve effectively. To achieve this important outcome, clinical activities should expose the learner to realistic clinical problems of increasing complexity.

Many nurse educators and nursing students believe that problem solving is synonymous with *critical thinking* (Ignatavicius, 2004; Ironside, 1999). However, the ability to solve clinical problems is insufficient for professional nursing practice because it focuses on the solution or outcome instead of a more complete understanding of a situation in context, derived from a deep understanding of the patient (Ironside, 1999).

Critical Thinking.   Critical thinking is an important outcome of nursing education. Early emphasis on developing critical thinking skills was stimulated by National League for Nursing Accrediting Commission (NLNAC) criteria for accreditation of nursing education programs. Programs accredited by the NLNAC are still expected to document evidence that their curricula provide for attainment of critical thinking skills, but it is no longer an accreditation standard, and it is not a specified standard for accreditation by the Commission on Collegiate Nursing Education (CCNE) (CCNE, 2003; Ignatavicius, 2004; NLNAC, 2005). Most employers of new nursing graduates, however, expect them to have this competency. A recent study of trends in professional nursing education programs revealed that critical thinking was expected to receive less emphasis in the future. This finding suggested that either nurse educators have incorporated critical thinking into curricula so well that they see no need for continued emphasis, that past emphasis on critical thinking had been driven by external forces, or that nurse educators perceive the need to *develop* rather than *teach* critical thinking skills (Speziale & Jacobson, 2005).

Many definitions of critical thinking exist, and the faculty must agree on a definition that is appropriate for a given program to provide direction for teaching and evaluating this outcome as well as communicating the construct effectively to students (Ignatavicius, 2004; Ironside, 1999; O'Sullivan, Blevins-Stephens, Smith, & Vaughn-Wrobel, 1997). One useful definition describes critical thinking as a process used to determine a course of action, involving collecting appropriate data, analyzing the validity and utility of the information, evaluating multiple lines of reasoning, and coming to valid conclusions (Beeken, Dale, Enos, & Yarbrough, 1997). It is also described as purposeful, outcome directed, and evidence based (Alfaro-LeFevre, 2004).

Although most educators would classify critical thinking as a knowledge outcome, some definitions of critical thinking characterize it as a composite of attitudes, knowledge, and skills. It involves the ability to seek and analyze truth systematically and with an open mind as well as attitudinal dimensions of self-confidence, maturity, and inquisitiveness (Dexter et al., 1997). Critical thinking requires habits of the mind such as reflective thinking, clinical reasoning, and clinical judgment (Alfaro-LeFevre, 2004). Clinical learning activities help learners to develop discipline-specific critical thinking skills as they observe, participate in, and evaluate nursing care in an increasingly complex and uncertain health care environment.

Decision Making.   Professional nursing practice requires nurses to make decisions about patients, staff members, and the clinical environment. The decision-making process involves gathering, analyzing, weighing, and valuing information in order to choose the best course of action from among a number of alternatives. Selecting the best alternative in terms of its relative benefits and consequences is a rational decision. However, nurses rarely know all possible alternatives, benefits, and risks; thus, clinical decision making usually involves some degree of uncertainty. Decisions are also influenced by an individual's values and biases and by cultural norms, which affect the way the individual perceives and analyzes the situation. In nursing, decision making is mutual and participatory with patients and staff members, so that the decisions are more likely to be accepted. Clinical education should involve learners in many realistic decision-making opportunities to produce this outcome.

Skills

Skills are another important outcome of clinical learning. Nurses must possess adequate psychomotor, interpersonal, and organizational skills to practice effectively in an increasingly complex health care environment. Skills often have cognitive and attitudinal dimensions, but the skill outcomes that must be produced by clinical teaching typically focus on the performance component.

Psychomotor Skills.   Psychomotor skills are integral to nursing practice, and deficiency in these skills among new graduates often leads to criticism of nursing education programs. Psychomotor skills enable nurses to perform effectively in action situations that require neuromuscular coordination. These skills are purposeful, complex, movement-oriented activities that involve an overt physical response. The term *skill* in this context refers to the ability to carry out physical movements efficiently and effectively, with speed and accuracy. Therefore, psychomotor skill is more than the capability to perform; it includes the ability to perform proficiently, smoothly, and consistently, under varying conditions and within appropriate time limits. Psychomotor skill learning requires practice with feedback to refine the performance until the desired outcome is achieved. Thus, clinical learning activities should include plentiful opportunities for practice of psychomotor skills with knowledge of results to facilitate the skill learning process.

Interpersonal Skills.   Interpersonal skills are used throughout the nursing process to assess patient and family needs, plan and implement care, evaluate the outcomes of care, and record and disseminate information. These skills include communication abilities, therapeutic use of self, and using the teaching process. Interpersonal skills involve knowledge of human behavior and social systems, but there also is a motor component largely comprising verbal behavior, such as speaking and writing, and nonverbal behavior, such as facial expression, body posture and movement, and touch. To encourage development of these outcomes, clinical learning activities should provide opportunities for students to form therapeutic relationships with patients; to develop collaborative relationships with health professionals; to document patient information, plans of care, care given, and evaluation results; and to teach patients, family members, and staff members, individually and in groups.

Organizational Skills.   Nurses need organizational and time management skills to practice competently in a complex environment. In clinical practice, students learn how to set priorities, manage conflicting expectations, and sequence their work to perform efficiently. One organizational skill that has become an important job expectation for professional nurses is delegation. In most health care settings, patient care is provided by a mix of licensed and unlicensed assistive personnel, and professional nurses must know how to delegate various aspects of patient care to others (Derickson & Caputi, 2004). Nurses need to know both the theory and skill of delegation—what to delegate, to whom, and under what circumstances—and to understand the legal aspects of empowering another person to carry out delegated tasks (Derickson & Caputi; Thomas & Hume, 1998). However, students will not learn these skills unless they are given opportunities to practice them with faculty guidance. As discussed in Chapter 7, if clinical learning assignments focus exclusively on total patient care activities, students will not gain enough experience in carrying out this delegation responsibility to perform it competently as graduates (Derickson & Caputi). Delegation skills are expected to receive greater emphasis in professional nursing education programs in the future (Speziale & Jacobson, 2005)

Depending on the level of the learner (e.g., graduate or undergraduate student, staff nurse), clinical activities also provide opportunities for learners to develop leadership and management skills. These skills include the ability to manage the care of a group of patients, to evaluate the performance of self and others, and to manage one's own career development (Derickson & Caputi, 2004; Sullivan & Decker, 2001; Yoder-Wise, 2003).

Attitudes and Values

Clinical learning also produces important affective outcomes—beliefs, values, attitudes, and dispositions that are essential elements of professional nursing practice. Affective outcomes represent the humanistic and ethical dimensions of nursing. Professional nurses are expected to hold and act on certain values with regard to patient care, such as respect for the individual's right to choose and the confidentiality of patient information. The values of professional nursing are expressed in the American Nurses Association *Code of Ethics for Nurses* (2001), and the nursing faculty should introduce the *Code* early in any nursing education program and reinforce its values by planning clinical learning activities that help students to develop them.

Additionally, nurses must be able to use the processes of moral reasoning, values clarification, and values inquiry. In an era of rapid knowledge and technology growth, nursing education programs also must produce graduates who are lifelong learners, committed to their own continued professional development.

Professional socialization is the process through which nurses and nursing students develop a sense of self as members of the profession, internalizing the norms and values of nursing in their own behavior. Professional socialization occurs at every level of nursing education: in initial preparation for nursing, when entering into the work setting as a new graduate, when returning to school for an advanced degree, and when changing roles within nursing.

Students are socialized into the role of professional nurse in the clinical setting, where accountability is demanded and the consequences of choices and actions are readily apparent. The clinical setting provides opportunities for students to develop, practice, and test these affective outcomes. Clinical education should expose students to strong role models, including nursing faculty members and practicing nurses, who demonstrate a commitment to professional values, and should provide value development opportunities that serve to socialize students to the profession (Weis & Schank, 2002).

Cultural Competence

Although the previous discussion classifies outcomes either as knowledge, skill, or attitude, some outcomes of clinical learning are not easily categorized. One example is cultural competence, an outcome that includes elements of knowledge, skill, and attitude. Several related terms have been used to refer to different variations of this outcome. Kleinman, Frederickson, and Lundy (2004) defined these terms as follows:

- *Cultural awareness:* the recognition that people live within some cultural context, both inherited and experiential, that is particular to their group.

- *Cultural sensitivity:* the belief that attention to the cultural contexts within which patients live influences patient care and promotes beneficial patient outcomes.

- *Cultural competence:* knowledge about an individual patient's cultural affiliations and the skill necessary to integrate them into the patient's care.

The population of the United States is becoming increasingly multicultural. If current population trends continue, by the year 2020 the percentage of Americans of European descent will fall from the 75% reported in the 2000 census to 53%. The population of Americans of Asian and Hispanic descent is expected to triple, and Black Americans are projected to double in number. To respond competently to these demographic changes, nursing students must be prepared to deal with diversity in all of its forms (Speziale & Jacobson, 2005). "Quality health care and cultural competency are correlated. In other words, providing the best nursing care is part of being culturally competent, and vice versa" (Johnson, 2005, p. 53).

The development of this outcome begins with awareness of cultural diversity and specific knowledge about cultural values, beliefs, rules, and traditions of the nurse's own culture as well as the patient's, and progresses to appreciating the similarities and differences between the nurse's and patients' cultures. Promoting culturally competent care is a priority in nursing and nursing education (Campinha-Bacote, 1998, 1999; Sutherland, 2004). Therefore, clinical teachers should plan learning activities that will challenge learners to explore cultural differences and to develop culturally appropriate responses to patient needs.

UNINTENDED OUTCOMES

Although nurse educators usually have the intended outcomes in mind when they design clinical learning activities, those activities may produce positive or negative unintended outcomes as well. Positive unintended outcomes include career choices that students and new graduate nurses make when they have clinical experiences in various settings. Exposure to a wide variety of clinical specialties stimulates learners to evaluate their own desires and competence to practice in those areas and allows them to make realistic career choices. For example, nursing students who do not have clinical learning activities in an operating room are unlikely to choose perioperative nursing as a specialty. However, if students participate in clinical activities in the operating room, some will realize that they are well suited to practice nursing in this area, while others will decide that perioperative nursing is not for them. In either case, students will have a realistic basis for their career choices.

Clinical learning activities can produce negative unintended outcomes as well. Nurse educators often worry that students will learn bad practice habits from observing other nurses in the clinical environment. Often, students are taught to perform skills, to document care, or to organize their work according to the instructor's preferences or to school or agency policy. However, students may observe staff members in the clinical setting who adapt skills, documentation, and organization of work to fit the unique needs of patients or the environment. Students often imitate the behaviors they observe, including taking shortcuts while performing skills, such as omitting steps that the teacher may believe are important to produce safe, effective outcomes. The power of role models to influence students' behavior and attitudes should not be underestimated. However, the clinical teacher should be careful not to label the teacher's way as good and all other ways as bad. Instead, the teacher should encourage learners to discuss the differences in practice habits that they have observed and to evaluate them in terms of theory or principle.

Another negative unintended outcome of clinical learning may be academic dishonesty. Academic dishonesty is intentional participation in deceptive practices such as lying, cheating, or false representation regarding one's academic work. Clinical teachers often try to instill the traditional health care cultural value that good nurses do not make errors. Even though the Institute of Medicine's report on health care errors (Kohn, Corrigan, & Donaldson 2000) has caused growing concern about patient safety and the need to prevent errors, a standard of perfection is unrealistic for any practitioner, let alone nursing students and new staff members whose mistakes are an inherent part of learning new knowledge and skills. A teacher's emphasis on perfection in clinical practice may produce the unintended result of student dishonesty in order to avoid punishment for making mistakes (Gaberson, 1997). Punishment for mistakes, in the form of low grades or negative performance evaluations, is not effective in preventing future errors. The unintended result of punishment for mistakes may be that learners conceal errors; failure to report errors can have dangerous consequences for patients in clinical settings and also creates lost opportunities for learners to learn to correct and then prevent their mistakes (Kohn et al.).

SUMMARY

Outcomes of clinical teaching include knowledge, skills, and attitudes that are acquired through clinical teaching and learning. Current nursing education program accreditation criteria focus on evidence that meaningful outcomes of learning have been produced. The effectiveness of clinical teaching can be judged on the extent to which it produces intended learning outcomes.

Clinical learning activities should focus on the development of *knowledge* that cannot be acquired in the classroom or other learning settings. In clinical practice, knowledge is applied to practice. In addition to understanding specific information, knowledge outcomes include cognitive skill in problem solving, critical thinking, and decision making. *Problem solving* ability is an important outcome of clinical teaching. Problems related to patients or the health care environment typically are unique, complex, and ambiguous, and often require new methods of reasoning and problem-solving strategies. *Critical thinking* is a process used to determine a course of action after collecting appropriate data, analyzing the validity and utility of the information, evaluating multiple lines of reasoning, and coming to valid conclusions. Critical thinking is facilitated by attitudinal dimensions of self-confidence, maturity, and inquisitiveness. Clinical learning activities help learners to develop discipline-specific critical thinking skills as they observe, participate in, and evaluate nursing care. *Decision making* involves gathering, analyzing, weighing, and valuing information to choose the best course of action from among a number of alternatives. Because nurses rarely know all possible alternatives, benefits, and risks, clinical decision making usually involves some degree of uncertainty. Clinical education should involve learners in realistic situations that require them to make decisions about patients, staff members, and the clinical environment in order to produce this outcome.

Skills are another important outcome of clinical learning. Many skills have cognitive and attitudinal dimensions, but clinical teaching typically focuses on the performance component. *Psychomotor skills* are purposeful, complex, movement-oriented activities that involve an overt physical response requiring neuromuscular coordination. Psychomotor skill includes the ability to perform proficiently, smoothly, and consistently, under varying conditions and within appropriate time limits. *Interpersonal skills* are used to assess client needs, to plan and implement patient care, to evaluate the outcomes of care, and to record and disseminate information. These skills include communication, therapeutic use of self, and teaching patients and others. Interpersonal skills involve knowledge of human behavior and social systems, but there also is a motor component largely comprising verbal and nonverbal behavior. Nurses need *organizational skills* to set priorities, manage conflicting expectations, and sequence their work to perform efficiently. Using *delegation skills* often is an important job expectation; nurses need to know what to delegate, to whom, and under what circumstances. Clinical learning activities provide opportunities for learners to develop leadership and *management skills*.

Clinical learning also produces important outcomes in *attitudes and values* that represent the humanistic and ethical dimensions of nursing. Professional nurses are expected to hold and act on certain values with regard to patient care and to use the processes of moral reasoning, values clarification, and values inquiry. These values are developed and internalized through the process of professional socialization. In an era of rapid knowledge and technology growth, nursing education programs also must produce graduates who are lifelong learners, committed to their own continued professional development.

One example of an outcome that encompasses knowledge, skills, and attitudes is cultural competence. *Cultural competence* is the ability to provide care that fits the cultural beliefs and practices of patients. This outcome includes understanding and appreciating the similarities and differences between the nurse's and patients' cultures.

Clinical learning activities also produce positive and negative *unintended* outcomes. Exposure to a wide variety of clinical specialties stimulates learners to evaluate their own desires and competence to practice in those areas and allows them to make realistic career choices. However, observing various role models in the clinical environment may result in students' learning bad practice habits. The unintended result of a teacher's unrealistic emphasis on perfection in clinical practice may be that learners conceal errors, with potentially dangerous consequences.

REFERENCES

Alfaro-LeFevre, R. (2004). *Critical thinking and critical judgment: A practical approach* (3rd ed.). St. Louis: Elsevier Saunders.

American Association of Colleges of Nursing. (1996). *The essentials of master's education for advanced practice nursing.* Washington, DC: Author.

American Association of Colleges of Nursing. (1998). *The essentials of baccalaureate education for professional nursing practice.* Washington, DC: Author.

American Nurses Association. (2001). *Code of ethics for nurses with interpretive statements.* Silver Spring, MD: Author.

Beeken, J. E., Dale, M. L., Enos, M. F., & Yarbrough, S. (1997). Teaching critical thinking skills to undergraduate nursing students. *Nurse Educator, 22,* 37–39.

Boland, D. L. (2005). Developing curriculum: Frameworks, outcomes, and competencies. In D. M. Billings & J. A. Halstead (Eds.), *Teaching in nursing: A guide for faculty* (2nd ed., pp. 167–186). St. Louis: Elsevier Saunders.

Boswell, C., & Cannon, S. (2005). Too much material, too little time: I'm drowning as a novice faculty member. *Nursing Education Perspectives, 26,* 208.

Campinha-Bacote, J. (1998). Cultural diversity in nursing education: Issues and concerns. *Journal of Nursing Education, 37,* 3–4.

Campinha-Bacote, J. (1999). A model and instrument for addressing cultural competence in health care. *Journal of Nursing Education, 38,* 203–207.

Commission on Collegiate Nursing Education. (2003). *Standards for accreditation of baccalaureate and graduate nursing programs.* Retrieved June 26, 2006, from http://www.aacn.nche.edu/Accreditation/NewStandards.htm

Derickson, L. M., & Caputi, L. (2004). *Teaching the critical thinking skills of delegating and prioritizing.* In L. Caputi & L. Engelmann (Eds.), *Teaching nursing: The art and science* (pp. 681–695). Glen Ellyn, IL: College of DuPage Press.

Dexter, P., Applegate, M., Backer, J., Claytor, K., Keefer, J., & Norton, B., et al. (1997). A proposed framework for teaching and evaluating critical thinking in nursing. *Journal of Professional Nursing, 13,* 160–167.

Diekelmann, N. L., Ironside, P. M., & Gunn, J. (2005). Recalling the Curriculum Revolution: Innovation with research. *Nursing Education Perspectives, 26,* 70–77.

Dillard, N., Sitkberg, L., & Laidig, J. (2005). Curriculum development: An overview. In D. M. Billings & J. A. Halstead (Eds.), *Teaching in nursing: A guide for faculty* (2nd ed., pp. 89–102). St. Louis: Elsevier Saunders.

Gaberson, K. B. (1997). Academic dishonesty among nursing students. *Nursing Forum, 32,* 14–20.

Ignatavicius, D. (2004). An introduction to developing critical thinking in nursing students. In L. Caputi & L. Engelmann (Eds.), *Teaching nursing: The art and science* (pp. 622–633). Glen Ellyn, IL: College of DuPage Press.

Ironside, P. M. (1999). Thinking in nursing education: A student's experience learning to think. *Nursing and Health Care Perspectives, 20,* 238–242.

Iwasiw, C. L., Goldenberg, D., & Andrusyszyn, M. (2005). Developing philosophical approaches and formulating curriculum goals. In *Curriculum development in nursing education.* Boston: Jones and Bartlett.

Johnson, L. D. (2005, Winter). The role of cultural competency in eliminating health disparities. *Minority Nurse, 52–55.*

Kleiman, S., Frederickson, K., & Lundy, T. (2004). Using an eclectic model to educate students about cultural influences on the nurse-patient relationship. *Nursing Education Perspectives, 25,* 249–253.

Kohn, L., Corrigan, J., & Donaldson, M. (2000). *To err is human: Building a safer health system.* Washington, DC: National Academy Press, Institute of Medicine.

National Council of State Boards of Nursing. (2004). *Test plan for the National Council Licensure Examination for Registered Nurses.* Retrieved June 26, 2006, from http://www.ncsbn.org/pdfs/RNTestPlan_Apr04.pdf

National League for Nursing Accrediting Commission. (2005). *Accreditation manual with interpretive guidelines by program type for postsecondary and higher degree programs in nursing.* Retrieved June 26, 2006, from http://www.nlnac.org/manuals/NLNACManual2005.pdf

O'Sullivan, P. S., Blevins-Stephens, W. L., Smith, F. M., & Vaughn-Wrobel, B. (1997). Addressing the National League for Nursing critical thinking outcome. *Nurse Educator, 22,* 23–29.

Speziale, H. J. S., & Jacobson, L. (2005). Trends in nurse education programs 1998–2008. *Nursing Education Perspectives, 26,* 230–235.

Sullivan, E., & Decker, P. J. (2001). *Effective leadership and management in nursing* (5th ed.). Upper Saddle River, NJ: Prentice Hall.

Sutherland, L. (2004). Teaching students from culturally diverse backgrounds. In L. Caputi & L. Engelmann (Eds.), *Teaching nursing: The art and science* (pp. 446–467). Glen Ellyn, IL: College of DuPage Press.

Thomas, S., & Hume, G. (1998). Delegation competencies: Beginning practitioners' reflections. *Nurse Educator, 23,* 38–41.

Weis, D., & Schank, M. J. (2002). Professional values: Key to professional development. *Journal of Professional Nursing, 18,* 271–275.

Yoder-Wise, P. S. (2003). *Leading and managing in nursing* (3rd ed.). St. Louis: Mosby.

Chapter 3

Preparing for Clinical Learning Activities

Nurse educators should consider a number of factors in preparing for clinical learning activities. Equipping students to enter the clinical setting must be balanced with preparing staff members for the presence of learners in a service setting and by respect for the needs of patients. This chapter describes the roles and responsibilities of faculty members, staff members, and others involved in clinical teaching and suggests methods of preparing students and staff members for clinical learning activities. Strategies for selecting clinical learning activities are discussed in Chapter 7.

UNDERSTANDING THE CONTEXT FOR CLINICAL LEARNING ACTIVITIES

To begin preparations for clinical teaching and learning, nurse educators should reflect on the context in which these activities take place. Teachers and learners use an established health care setting for a learning environment, thus creating a temporary system within a permanent system. What are the effects of clinical teaching as a temporary system?

Since the early 1900s, basic preparation for professional nursing has evolved from service-based training and apprenticeship into academic educational programs in institutions of higher learning. As a result of this service–education separation, the clinical teacher and students who enter a clinical setting for learning activities often are regarded as strangers or guests in the permanent social system of a health care agency. They participate in the activities of the clinical system and attempt to follow the norms of its culture, but they are not a constant presence (Case & Oermann, 2004; Paterson, 1997).

The clinical teacher and students in an academic nursing education program comprise a temporary system within the permanent culture of the clinical setting. Similarly, a staff development instructor and orientees may represent a temporary system. A temporary system is a set of individuals who work together on a complex task over a limited period of time. In contrast, staff members in the clinical agency have long-term membership in a permanent system with well-defined roles and identities. Although many clinical teachers view themselves as professional colleagues of nursing staff members, they are at the same time alienated from the permanent structure of the clinical agency (Paterson, 1997). Even if they are employed by the agency as staff members on a casual or part-time basis, in addition to their academic positions, faculty members enact a different role in that agency when they are guiding the clinical learning activities of students.

Consequences for clinical teachers and their students of being a temporary system in the clinical setting include territoriality, defensiveness, separateness, and inadequate communication. Both permanent and temporary systems establish territorial boundaries that are communicated through verbal and nonverbal behavior. Teachers often coach students to ask permission before using property, to appear pleasant and grateful, and to relinquish a patient's chart if it is requested by a physician or a staff nurse. Packford and Polifroni (1992) depicted the clinical teacher as straddling the gap between academia and service. In this context, clinical teachers function as diplomats and negotiators with staff members while serving as gatekeepers, buffers, and protectors of students. Often, the effect on students of these gatekeeping and protecting functions is to stifle learning. Because of faculty members' desire for credibility and acceptance by staff members, they tend to minimize students' risk taking in an effort to prevent mistakes (Packford & Polifroni, 1992).

Students often are viewed by the nursing staff as the teacher's responsibility, and although students may be encouraged to use staff nurses as resources, both students and staff may avoid this contact. Teachers and nursing staff members may exhibit defensiveness when their competence and professional identities are criticized by members of the other system. The separateness of the two systems may be evident in the lack of extensive interactions between them, and nursing staff members and clinical teachers may fail to communicate essential information to each other. To overcome these negative consequences, clinical teachers often attempt to court the staff by being responsive, avoiding confrontations about patient care, and monitoring students closely to minimize errors that might aggravate staff. Some of these consequences may be avoided by a simple measure such as regular meetings between teachers and nurse managers (Paterson, 1997).

Although clinical teachers and nursing students are guests in the health care environment, they also are a vital resource to a health care agency. Nursing students represent potential future employees of that organization, and most health care administrators and managers view the presence of nursing students in the facility as a recruitment opportunity (Case & Oermann, 2004). Positive clinical learning experiences may encourage nursing students to consider future employment in that agency, and nursing staff members who nurture the development of students can have a powerful influence on such a choice.

In a sense, the role of the clinical teacher is that of culture broker, in which the teacher interprets the norms of the clinical culture to the students and the norms of the academic culture to the staff members. The focus of the health care agency is on delivery of quality patient care resulting in measurable positive outcomes; the focus of the educational institution is on the learning needs of the students (Hunsberger et al., 2000). The clinical and management staffs of the health care agency are responsible for providing quality care to patients, as specified in standards of the Joint Commission for Accreditation of Healthcare Organizations. Many staff members, however, are unaware of or misinterpret this standard; they expect nursing students to participate fully in all unit activities, assume responsibility for patient care, take the same kinds of patient assignments, and complete the same patient care tasks as do staff members. They may recall their own clinical education as being more rigorous than the contemporary clinical activities that they witness (Case & Oermann, 2004); communicating those perceptions to nursing students can produce self-doubt, discouragement, and dissatisfaction among these novices. The teacher as culture broker must allow students to experience the real world of clinical nursing, and at the same time, communicate to staff members that trends and current issues in nursing education mean that "it's not your mother's nursing school." Keeping clinical agency staff members, managers, and administrators informed about the nature of contemporary nursing education and keeping students updated on current challenges and priorities in the health care environment will help to integrate students more effectively into the real world of clinical nursing.

SELECTING CLINICAL SETTINGS

Clinical teachers may have sole responsibility for selecting the settings in which clinical learning activities occur, or their input may be sought by those who make these decisions. In either case, selection of clinical sites should be based on important criteria such as compatibility of school and agency philosophy, type of practice model used, availability of opportunities to meet learning objectives, geographical location, availability of role models, and physical resources (Stokes & Kost, 2004).

In some areas, selection of appropriate clinical settings may be difficult because of competition among several nursing programs, and nursing programs typically must contract with a variety of agencies to provide adequate learning opportunities for students. Using a large number of clinical sites increases the time and energy required for teachers to develop relationships with staff, to obtain necessary information about agencies, and to develop and maintain competence to practice in diverse settings.

Selection Criteria

Nurse educators should conduct a careful assessment of potential clinical sites before selecting those that will be used. Faculty members who also are employed in clinical agencies may provide some of the necessary information, and teachers who have instructed students in an agency can provide ongoing input into its continued suitability as a practice site. Assessment of potential clinical agencies should address the following criteria (Case & Oermann, 2004):

• *Opportunity to achieve learning outcomes.* Are sufficient opportunities available to allow learners to achieve learning objectives? For example, if planning, implementing, and evaluating preoperative teaching is an important course objective, the average preoperative patient census must be sufficient to permit learners to practice these skills. If the objectives require learners to practice direct patient care, does the agency allow this, or will learners only be permitted to observe? Will learners from other educational programs also be present in the clinical environment at the same time? If so, how much competition for the same learning opportunities is anticipated?

• *Level of the learner.* If the learners are undergraduate students at the beginning level of the curriculum, the agency must provide ample opportunity to practice basic skills. Graduate students need learning activities that will allow them to develop advanced practice skills. Does the clinical agency permit graduate students to practice independently or under the guidance of a preceptor, without an on-site instructor? Are undergraduate students in a capstone course permitted to participate in clinical learning activities under the guidance of an appropriate staff member as preceptor, without the physical presence of a faculty member?

• *Degree of control by faculty.* Does the agency staff recognize the authority of the clinical teacher to plan appropriate learning activities for students, or do agency policies limit or prescribe the kinds and timing of student activities? Do agency personnel view learners as additions to the staff and expect them to provide service to patients, or do they acknowledge the role of students as learners?

• *Compatibility of philosophies.* Are the philosophies of clinical agency and educational program compatible? For example, the philosophy of a school of nursing emphasizes patients' right to self-determination, but the agency within which students are to be placed for perioperative nursing clinical practice routinely suspends patients' "do not resuscitate" advanced directives when they are scheduled for surgery. In this example, the faculty member might wish to seek another agency whose philosophy of care is more compatible with that of the school.

• *Availability of role models for students.* As discussed in Chapter 2, students often imitate the behaviors they observe in staff nurses. Are the agency staff members positive role models for students and new staff nurses? If learners are graduate students who are learning advanced practice roles, are strong, positive role models available to serve as preceptors and mentors? Is staffing adequate to permit staff members to interact with students?

• *Geographical location.* Although geographical location of the clinical agency usually is not the most important selection criterion, often it is a crucial factor when a large number of clinical agencies must be used. Travel time between the campus and clinical settings for faculty and students must be considered, especially if learning activities are scheduled in both settings on the same day. Is travel to the agency via public transportation possible and safe, especially if faculty and students must travel in the evening or at night? Are public transportation schedules convenient—do they allow students and faculty to arrive at the agency in time for the scheduled start of activities, and do they permit a return trip to campus or home without excessive wait times? Does the value of available learning opportunities at the agency outweigh the disadvantages of travel time and cost?

• *Physical facilities.* Are physical facilities such as conference space, locker room or other space to store personal belonging, cafeteria or other dining facility, library and other reference materials, and parking available for use by clinical teachers and students?

• *Staff relationships with teachers and learners.* Do staff members respond positively to the presence of students? Will the staff members cooperate with teachers in selecting appropriate learning activities and participate in orientation activities for faculty and students?

• *Orientation needs.* Some clinical agencies require faculty members to attend scheduled orientation sessions before they take students into the clinical setting. The time required for such orientation must be considered when selecting clinical agencies. If faculty members are also employed in the agency as casual or per diem staff, this orientation requirement may be waived. Are any parts of the orientation able to be completed without being present in the agency, such as online or self-study?

• *Opportunity for interdisciplinary activities.* Are there opportunities for learners to practice as members of an interdisciplinary health care team? Will learners have contact with other health care practitioners such as physical therapists, pharmacists, nutritionists, respiratory therapists, social workers, infection control personnel, and physicians?

• *Agency requirements.* Unless the educational program and the clinical facility are parts of the same organization, a legal contract or agreement usually must be negotiated to permit students and faculty to use the agency as a clinical teaching site. Such contracts or agreements typically specify requirements such as school and individual liability insurance; competence in cardiopulmonary resuscitation; professional licensure for faculty, graduate students, and RN-BSN students; immunization and other health requirements; dress code; use of name tags or identification badges; requirements for student drug testing, and requirements for criminal background checks for students and clinical teachers. Sufficient time must be allowed before the anticipated start of clinical activities to negotiate the contract and for faculty and students to meet the requirements. Faculty members usually must have current unencumbered professional nursing licenses for each state in which they instruct in the clinical area, unless the clinical agencies are located in states that have adopted the Nurse Licensure Compact (National Council of State Boards of Nursing, n.d.) and the faculty member also is licensed in one of those states.

• *Agency licensure and accreditation.* Accreditation requirements for educational programs may specify that clinical learning activities take place in accredited health care organizations. If the agency must be licensed to provide certain health services, it is appropriate to verify current licensure before selecting that agency as a clinical site.

• *Costs.* In addition to travel expenses, there may be other costs associated with use of an agency for clinical learning activities. Any fees charged to schools for use of the agency or other anticipated expense to the educational program and to individual clinical teachers and students should be assessed.

PREPARATION OF FACULTY

When selection of the clinical site or sites is complete, the nurse educator must prepare for the teaching and learning activities that will take place there. Areas of preparation that must be addressed include clinical competence, familiarity with the clinical environment, and orientation to the agency.

Clinical Competence

Clinical competence has been documented as an essential characteristic of effective clinical teachers (Stokes & Kost, 2004). It includes theoretical knowledge of and expert clinical skills and judgement in the practice area in which teaching occurs (Oermann, 1996; Oermann & Gaberson, 2006).

Standards for accreditation and state approval of nursing education programs may require nurse faculty members to have advanced clinical preparation in graduate nursing programs in the clinical specialty area in which they are assigned to teach. In addition, faculty members should have sufficient clinical experience in the specialty area in which they teach. The combination of academic preparation and professional work experience supports the teacher's credibility and confidence and is particularly important for faculty members who will provide direct, on-site guidance of students in the clinical area. Students often identify the ability to demonstrate nursing care in the clinical setting as an essential skill of an effective clinical instructor (Case & Oermann, 2004; Krafft, 1998; Stokes & Kost, 2004).

Clinical teachers should maintain current clinical knowledge through participation in continuing education and practice experience. Teachers in academic settings who have a concurrent faculty practice or joint appointment in a clinical agency are able to maintain their clinical competence by this means, especially if they practice in the same specialty area and clinical agency in which they teach (Krafft, 1998).

Familiarity With Clinical Environment

If the clinical teacher is entering a new clinical area, he or she may ask to work with the staff for a few days prior to returning to the site with students. During this time the teacher can practice using equipment that may be unfamiliar and become familiar with the agency environment, policies, and procedures. If working with the staff is not possible, the teacher should at least observe activities in the clinical area to discern the characteristics of the patient population; the usual schedule and pace of activities; the types of learning opportunities available to develop desired knowledge, skills, and attitudes; the diversity of health care professionals in the agency; and the presence of other learners (Case & Oermann, 2004).

Orientation

As previously mentioned, a clinical agency may require faculty members whose students use the facility to attend an orientation program. Orientation sessions vary in length from several hours to a day or more and typically include introductions to administrators, managers, and staff development instructors; clarification of policies such as whether students may administer intravenous medications; review of documentation procedures; and safety procedures. Faculty members may be asked to demonstrate competent operation of equipment, such as infusion pumps, that their students will be using or to submit evidence that they have met the same competency standards that are required of nursing staff members.

PREPARATION OF CLINICAL AGENCY STAFF

Preparation of the clinical agency staff usually begins with the teacher's initial contact with the agency as a basis for negotiating an agreement or contract between the educational program and the agency. Establishing an effective working relationship with the nursing staff is an important responsibility of the teacher. Ideally, nursing staff members would be eager to work with the faculty member to help students meet their learning goals. Indeed, in academic health centers and other teaching institutions, participation in education of learners from many health care disciplines is a normal job expectation. In reality, however, some staff members enjoy working with students more than others do. Because teachers usually cannot choose which staff members will be involved with students, it is important for the teacher to communicate to all staff members information about role expectations, the level of the learners' education and experience, the purpose and desired learning outcomes, the need for positive role modeling, and the role of staff members in evaluation.

Clarification of Roles

As previously discussed, staff members often expect the instructor take complete responsibility for the students; this expectation may extend to the instructor being responsible for the care of patients with whom students are assigned to work. Many clinical teachers remark that if they have 10 students and each student is assigned 2 patients, the instructor is responsible for 30 individuals. These role expectations are both unrealistic and unfair to all involved parties.

Although the clinical teacher is ultimately responsible for student learning, students have much to gain from close working relationships with staff members. Staff members can serve as useful role models of nursing practice in the real world; students can observe how staff members must adapt their practice to fit the demands of a complex, ever-changing clinical environment. At the same time, staff members often are stimulated and motivated by students' questions and the current information that they can share. The presence of students in the clinical environment often reinforces staff members' own competence and expertise, and many nurses enjoy sharing their knowledge and skill with novices. Clinical teachers, therefore, should encourage staff members to participate in the instruction of learners, within guidelines that teachers and staff members develop jointly. Students should be encouraged to use staff members as resources for their learning, especially when they have questions that relate to specific patients for whom the staff members are responsible.

An important point of role clarification is that the responsibility for patient care remains with staff members of the clinical agency, as mentioned earlier. If a student is assigned learning activities related to a specific patient, a staff member is always assigned the overall responsibility for that patient's care. Students are accountable for their own actions, but the staff member should collaborate with the student to ensure that patient needs are met. Staff members may give reports about patient status and needs to students who are assigned to work with those patients; students should be encouraged to ask questions of staff members about specific patient care requirements, to share ideas about patient care, and to report changes in patient condition, problems, tasks that they will not be able to complete, and the need for assistance with tasks (Case & Oermann, 2004).

Role expectation guidelines should be discussed with staff members and managers. When mutual understanding is achieved, the guidelines may be written and posted or distributed to relevant personnel and students.

Level of Learners

Staff members can have reasonable expectations of learner performance if they are informed of the students' levels of education and experience. Beginning students and novice staff members will need more guidance; staff members working with these learners should expect frequent questions and requests for assistance. More experienced learners may need less assistance with tasks but more guidance on problem solving and clinical decision making. Sharing this information with staff members allows them to plan their time accordingly and to anticipate student needs.

It is especially important for faculty members to tell agency personnel what specific tasks or activities learners are permitted and not permitted to do. This decision may be guided by nursing education program or agency policy, the curriculum sequence, or by the specific focus of the learning activities on any given day. For example, during one scheduled clinical session an instructor may want students to practice therapeutic use of self through interviewing and active listening, without relying on physical care tasks. The instructor should share this information with the staff members and ask them to avoid involving students in physical care on that day.

Learning Outcomes

The overall purpose and desired outcomes of the clinical learning activities should be communicated to staff members. As previously noted, knowledge of the specific objectives for a clinical session permits staff members to collaborate with the teacher in facilitating learning. If students have the specific learning objective of administering intramuscular injections, staff members can be asked to notify the teacher if any patient needs an injection that day so that the student can take advantage of that learning opportunity.

Knowledge of the learning objectives allows staff members to suggest appropriate learning activities even if the teacher is unable to anticipate the need. For example, an elderly patient who is confused may be admitted to the nursing unit; the staff nurse who is aware that students are focusing on nursing interventions to achieve patient safety might suggest that a student be assigned to work with this patient.

Need for Positive Role Modeling

The need for staff members to be positive role models for learners is a sensitive but important issue. As discussed in Chapter 2, teachers often worry that students will learn bad practice habits from experienced nurses who may take shortcuts when giving care. When discussing this issue with staff members, instructors should avoid implying that the only right way to perform skills is the teacher's way. Instead, the teacher might ask staff members to point out when they are omitting steps from procedures and to discuss with learners the rationale for those actions. In this way, staff nurses can model "how to think like a nurse," a valuable learning opportunity for nursing students (Ironside, 1999).

Asking staff nurses to be aware of the behaviors that they model for students and seeking their collaboration in fostering students' professional role development is an important aspect of preparing agency staff to work with learners. To accomplish this goal, instructors need to establish mutually respectful, trusting relationships with staff member and to sustain dialogue about role modeling over a period of time.

The Role of Staff Members in Evaluation

Agency staff members have important roles in evaluating learner performance. The clinical performance of learners must be evaluated formatively and summatively. *Formative evaluation* takes the form of feedback to the student during the learning process; its purpose is to provide information to be used by the learner to improve performance. *Summative evaluation* occurs at the end of the learning process; its outcome is a judgment about the worth or value of the learning outcomes (Oermann & Gaberson, 2006). Summative evaluations usually result in academic grades or personnel decisions such as promotions or merit pay increases.

Teachers should explain carefully their expectations about the desired involvement of staff members in evaluating student performance. Agency personnel have an important role in formative evaluation by communicating with teachers and learners about student performance. Because staff members often are in close contact with students during clinical activities, their observations of student performance are valuable (Case & Oermann, 2004). Staff members should be encouraged to report to the teacher any concerns that they may have about student performance as well as observations of exemplary performance. At the same time, they should feel free to praise students or to point out any errors they may have made or suggestions for improving performance. Immediate, descriptive feedback is necessary for learners to improve their performance, and often staff members are better able than teachers to provide this information to students.

However, it is the teacher's responsibility to make summative evaluation decisions. Staff members should know that they are an important source of data on student performance and that their input is valued, but that ultimately it is the clinical teacher who certifies competence or assigns a grade.

PREPARING THE LEARNERS

Students need cognitive, psychomotor, and affective preparation for clinical learning activities. It is the clinical teacher's responsibility to assist students with such preparation as well as to assess its adequacy before students enter the clinical area. Students also need an orientation to the setting in which clinical learning activities will occur, and specific preparation for the first day in a new setting.

Cognitive Preparation

General prerequisite knowledge for clinical learning includes information about the learning outcomes, the clinical agency, and the roles of teacher, student, and staff member. Additionally, in some nursing programs, students are able to prepare ahead of time for each clinical learning session. This preparation may include one or more of the following: gathering information from patient records; interviewing a patient; assessing patient needs; performing physical assessment; reviewing relevant pathophysiology, nursing, nutrition, and pharmacology textbooks; and completing written assignments such as a patient assessment or plan of care. In other programs students complete these types of learning activities during and following their clinical learning activities.

Teachers should ensure that the expected cognitive preparations for clinical learning do not carry more importance than the actual clinical learning activities themselves. That is, learning should be expected to occur during the clinical learning activities as well as during preclinical planning. If students receive their assignments in advance of the scheduled clinical activity, they can reasonably be expected to review relevant textbook information and to anticipate potential patient problems and needs. If circumstances permit a planning visit to the clinical agency, the student may meet and interview the patient and review the patient record. However, requiring extensive written assignments to be completed before the actual clinical activity implies that learning takes place only before the student enters the clinical area. Students cannot be expected to formulate a reasonable plan of care before assessing the patient's physical, psychosocial, and cultural needs; this assessment may begin before the actual clinical activity, but it usually comprises a major part of the student's activity in the clinical setting. Thus, preclinical planning should focus on preparations for the learning that will take place in clinical practice. For example, the teacher may require students to formulate a tentative nursing diagnosis from available patient information, to formulate a plan for collecting additional data to support or refute this diagnosis, and to plan tentative nursing interventions based on the diagnosis. A more extensive written assignment submitted after the clinical activity may require students to evaluate the appropriateness of the diagnosis and the effectiveness of the nursing interventions.

Additionally, because students often copy information from textbooks (or, regrettably, from other students) to complete such requirements, written assignments submitted before the actual clinical learning activity may not show evidence of critical thinking and problem solving, let alone comprehension and retention of the information. For example, some teachers require students to complete drug cards for each medication prescribed for a patient. Students often copy published pharmacologic information without attempting to retain this information and to think critically about why the medication was prescribed or how a particular patient might respond to it. A better approach is to ask students to reflect on the pharmacologic actions of prescribed drugs and to be prepared to discuss relevant nursing care implications, either individually with the instructor or in a group conference.

Psychomotor Preparation

Skill learning is an important outcome of clinical teaching. However, the length and number of clinical learning sessions are often limited in nursing education or new staff orientation programs. When learning complex skills, it is more efficient for students to practice the parts first in an environment such as a simulation center or skills laboratory, free from the demands of the actual practice setting. In such a setting, students can investigate and discover alternate ways of performing skills, and they can make errors and learn to correct them without fear of harming patients. Thus, students should have ample skill practice time before they enter the clinical area so that they are not expected to perform a skill for the first time in a fast-paced, demanding environment. It is the clinical teacher's responsibility to assure that students have developed the desired level of skill before entering the clinical setting.

Affective Preparation

Affective preparation of students includes strategies for managing their anxiety and for fostering confidence and positive attitudes about learning. Most students have some anxiety about clinical learning activities. Mild or moderate anxiety often serves to motivate students to learn, but excessive anxiety hinders concentration and interferes with learning (Arnold & Nieswiadomy, 1997). The role of the teacher in reducing the stress of clinical practice is discussed in more detail in Chapter 4. However, in preparation for clinical learning activities, teachers may employ strategies to identify students' fears and reduce their anxiety to a manageable level. A preclinical conference session might assess learners' specific concerns and assure students of the teacher's confidence in them, desire for their success, and availability for consultation and guidance during the clinical activities.

One example of an approach to reducing anxiety prior to clinical activities in a psychiatric setting was described by Arnold and Nieswiadomy (1997). In this study, students who participated in a structured communication exercise focused on identifying and discussing their anxiety about clinical activities showed significantly lower levels of anxiety on the first day of clinical practice than students who participated in a nonstructured question-and-answer session. However, for this strategy to be effective, students must be assured that revealing their fears and doubts will not influence their teacher's evaluation of their performance (Arnold & Nieswiadomy, 1997).

Orientation to the Clinical Agency

Like clinical teachers, students also need a thorough orientation to the clinical agency in which learning activities will take place. This orientation may take place before or on the first day of clinical activities. Staff members often assist the teacher in orienting students to the agency and helping them to feel welcome and comfortable in the new environment.

Orientation should include

- the geographical location of the agency;
- the physical setup of the specific unit where students will be placed;
- names, titles, and roles of personnel;
- location of areas such as restrooms, dining facilities, conference room, locker rooms, public telephones, and library;
- information about transportation and parking;
- agency and unit policies;
- daily schedules and routines;
- patient information documentation systems.

In addition, students need to have a phone number where they can be contacted in case of family emergency, know what procedures to follow in case of illness or other reason for absence on a clinical day, and understand the uniform or dress requirements.

Not all of this information needs to be presented on-site; some creative clinical teachers have developed audiovisual media, such as videotapes or slide-tape programs, that provide a vicarious tour of the facility. If the agency uses computer software to document patient information, the instructor may be able to acquire a copy of the program and make it available in the school's computer facility. Learners can be expected to review such media before coming to the clinical site.

Preparing for the First Day

Students almost always perceive the first day of clinical learning activities in a new setting as stressful; this is especially true of learners in their initial clinical nursing course (Admi, 1997). Students' first exposure to the clinical environment either can promote their independence as learners or foster dependence on the instructor due to fear. Clinical teachers should plan specific activities for the first day that will allow learners to become familiar with and comfortable in the clinical environment and at the same time alleviate their anxiety. These activities may include tours, conferences, games, and special assignments.

Even if learners have attended an agency orientation, it is helpful to take them on a tour of the specific areas they will use for learning activities, pointing out locations such as restrooms, drinking fountains, fire alarms and extinguishers, and elevators, stairwells, and emergency exits. The instructor should introduce learners to staff members by name and title. If students need agency-specific identification badges, parking permits, or passwords for use of the computer system, the teacher may make the necessary arrangements ahead of time or accompany students to the appropriate locations where these items can be acquired.

Special assignments may include review and discussion of patient records, practice of computer documentation, and a treasure hunt or scavenger hunt to help learners to locate typical items needed for patient care. Table 3.1 is an example of

TABLE 3.1   A Scavenger Hunt Activity

Anywhere General Hospital
Unit 2C

Work in pairs to search for the location of the items or areas listed below. Check them off as you find them.

❑ Locker room
❑ Restrooms
❑ Oxygen shut-off valves
❑ Fire alarms
❑ Fire extinguishers
❑ Emergency exits
❑ Assignment board
❑ Patient records
❑ Patient teaching materials
❑ Nurse Manager's office
❑ Medication dispensing cabinet
❑ Linen carts
❑ Kitchen
❑ Utility room
❑ Reference materials
❑ Conference room

---

a scavenger hunt activity used in orienting students to a medical-surgical unit of a hospital. Learners may be asked to observe patient care for a specified period of time, to interview a patient or family member, or to complete a short written assignment focused on documenting an observation.

These activities may be followed by a short group conference during which students are encouraged to discuss their impressions, experiences, and feelings. The teacher should review the roles of student, teacher, and staff members and should emphasize lines of communication. For example, students need to know who to ask for help and under what circumstances, that is, when to ask questions of staff members and when to seek assistance from the teacher. Handouts summarizing these expectations and requirements are useful because students can review them later when their anxiety is lower. If available in the clinical setting, this conference may take place in the dining facility to allow students to relax with refreshments away from patient care areas. The conference may conclude by making plans for the next day of clinical practice, including selecting assignments and discussing how learners should prepare for their learning activities. Selection of clinical assignments is discussed in detail in Chapter 7.

SUMMARY

This chapter described the roles and responsibilities of faculty, staff members, and others involved in clinical teaching and suggested strategies for preparing students and staff members for clinical learning.

The teacher and learners comprise a temporary system within the permanent culture of the clinical setting. Consequences for clinical teachers and their students of being a temporary system in the clinical setting include territoriality, defensiveness, separateness, and inadequate communication. Clinical teachers often function as diplomats and negotiators with staff members while serving as gatekeepers, buffers, and protectors of students. The effect of these gatekeeping and protecting functions may be to stifle learning. Some of these negative consequences may be avoided by establishing and maintaining good working relationships and regular communication between instructor and staff members. Clinical teachers should function as culture brokers to help integrate students more fully into the real world of nursing practice.

Settings for clinical learning should be selected carefully, based on important criteria such as compatibility of school and agency philosophy, type of practice model used, availability of opportunities to meet learning objectives, geographical location, availability of role models, and physical resources. Selection of appropriate clinical settings may be complicated by competition among several nursing programs for a limited number of agencies. Using multiple clinical sites increases the time and energy required for teachers to develop relationships with staff, obtain necessary information about agencies, and develop and maintain competence to practice in diverse settings. Specific criteria for assessing the suitability of potential clinical settings were discussed.

When clinical sites have been selected, educators must prepare for teaching and learning activities. Areas of preparation include clinical competence, familiarity with the clinical environment, and orientation to the agency. Clinical competence has been documented as an essential characteristic of effective clinical teachers and includes knowledge and expert skill and judgment in the clinical practice area in which teaching occurs. Teachers may maintain clinical competence through faculty practice, joint appointment in clinical agencies, and continuing nursing education activities. The teacher may become familiar with a new clinical setting by working with or observing the staff for a few days prior to returning to the site with students. The clinical agency may require faculty members to attend an orientation program that includes introductions to agency staff, clarification of policies concerning student activities, and review of skills and procedures.

Preparation of the clinical agency staff usually begins with the teacher's initial contact with the agency; establishing effective working relationships with the nursing staff yields important benefits for students. Roles of teacher, students, and staff members should be clarified so that staff members have guidelines for their participation in the instruction of learners. An important point of role clarification is that although students are accountable for their own actions, the responsibility for patient care remains with staff members of the clinical agency. Staff members also need to be aware of specific learning objectives, the level of the learner, the need for positive role modeling, and expectations concerning their role in evaluation student performance. Although staff members' feedback is valuable in formative evaluation, the teacher always is responsible for summative evaluation of learner performance.

Students need cognitive, psychomotor, and affective preparation for clinical learning activities. Cognitive preparation includes information about the learning objectives, the clinical agency, and the roles of teacher, student, and staff member. Students may be expected to prepare for each clinical learning session through reading, interviewing patients, and completing written assignments. However, requirements for extensive written assignments to be completed before the actual clinical activity may imply that learning takes place only before the student enters the clinical area.

The instructor has a responsibility to assess that students have the desired level of skill development before entering the clinical setting. When learning complex skills, it is more efficient for students to practice the parts first in a simulated setting such as a skills laboratory, free from the demands of the actual practice setting. Students should have ample skill practice time before they enter the clinical area so that they are not expected to perform a skill for the first time in a fast-paced, demanding environment.

Affective preparation of students includes strategies for managing their anxiety and for fostering confidence and positive attitudes about learning. Most students have some anxiety about clinical learning activities. Mild or moderate anxiety often serves to motivate students to learn, but excessive anxiety hinders concentration and interferes with learning. In preparation for clinical learning activities, teachers may employ strategies such as a structured preclinical conference to identify students' fears and reduce their anxiety to a manageable level.

Students also need a thorough orientation to the clinical agency in which learning activities will take place. This orientation should include information about the location and physical setup of the agency, relevant agency personnel, agency policies, daily schedules and routines, and procedures for responding to emergencies and for documenting patient information.

Students almost always perceive the first day of clinical learning activities in a new setting as stressful. Clinical teachers should plan specific activities for the first day that will allow learners to become familiar with and comfortable in the clinical environment and at the same time alleviate their anxiety. These activities include tours, conferences, games, and special assignments.

REFERENCES

Admi, H. (1997). Nursing students' stress during the initial clinical experience. *Journal of Nursing Education, 36,* 323–327.

Arnold, W. K., & Nieswiadomy, R. M. (1997). A structured communication exercise to reduce nursing students' anxiety prior to entering the psychiatric setting. *Journal of Nursing Education, 36,* 446–447.

Case, B., & Oermann, M. H. (2004). Teaching in a clinical setting. In L. Caputi & L. Engelmann (Eds.), *Teaching nursing: The art and science* (pp. 126–177). Glen Ellyn, IL: College of DuPage Press.

Hunsberger, M., Baumann, A., Lappan, J., Carter, N., Bowman, A., Goddard, P., et al. (2000). The synergism of expertise in clinical teaching: An integrative model for nursing education. *Journal of Nursing Education, 39,* 278–282.

Ironside, P. M. (1999). Thinking in nursing education: A student's experience learning to think. *Nursing and Health Care Perspectives, 20,* 238–242.

Krafft, S. K. (1998). Faculty practice: Why and how. *Nurse Educator, 23,* 45–48.

National Council of State Boards of Nursing. (n.d.). *Nurse licensure compact.* Retrieved June 26, 2006, from http://ncsbn.org/nlc/index.asp

Oermann, M. H. (1996). Research on teaching in the clinical setting. In K. R. Stevens (Ed.), *Review of research in nursing education* (Vol. VII, pp. 91–126). New York: National League for Nursing.

Oermann, M. H., & Gaberson, K. B. (2006). *Evaluation and testing in nursing education* (2nd ed.). New York: Springer Publishing.

Packford, S., & Polifroni, E. C. (1992). Role perceptions and role dilemmas of clinical nurse educators. In L. B. Welch (Ed.), *Perspectives on faculty roles in nursing education* (pp. 55–74). New York: Praeger.

Paterson, B. L. (1997). The negotiated order of clinical teaching. *Journal of Nursing Education, 36,* 197–205.

Stokes, L., & Kost, G. (2005). Teaching in the clinical setting. In D. M. Billings & J. A. Halstead (Eds.), *Teaching in nursing: A guide for faculty* (2nd ed., pp. 325–348). St. Louis: Elsevier Saunders.

Chapter 4

Clinical Teaching: Teacher, Student, and Models to Guide Teaching

Clinical practice provides an opportunity for students to acquire the knowledge needed for patient care, clinical judgment and critical thinking skills, a professional value system to guide their decision making in practice, and an array of technological skills. Students can learn about concepts, theories, and other types of knowledge in a classroom, from an online course, and in a simulation laboratory, but it is only in the practice setting where they begin to use that knowledge in caring for patients and are exposed to clinical situations that may not be the same as discussed in class or the literature. In clinical practice students develop their clinical judgment and other cognitive skills, and test their values with patients, families, and staff. The clinical activities in which students engage are critical for developing these competencies.

Planning the clinical activities and effectively guiding students in the practice setting require a teacher who is knowledgeable about the clinical practice area, is clinically competent, knows how to teach, relates effectively to students, and is enthusiastic about clinical teaching. The teacher also serves as a role model for students or selects clinicians who will model important professional behaviors and the role for which the student is preparing.

This chapter describes the characteristics of effective clinical teachers, stresses of students in clinical practice and of clinical teachers, the socialization of students through their clinical experiences, and various models for clinical teaching.

QUALITIES OF EFFECTIVE CLINICAL TEACHERS

There has been much research in nursing on characteristics and qualities of an effective clinical teacher, and some general principles can be drawn from this research. Findings of studies on effective clinical teaching in nursing are consistent with research in medical education and higher education in general. Every clinical teacher should be aware of qualities and behaviors that promote learning in the practice setting and ones that impede student learning.

Knowledge

Teachers in nursing as in any field need to have expertise in the *subject* they are teaching; clinical educators must be knowledgeable about the types of patient problems in the clinical setting and how to manage them, new technologies in patient care, and related research. Teachers must be up-to-date in the area of clinical practice in which they are working with students, especially when following the traditional model of clinical teaching in which the teacher is responsible for planning and guiding student learning in practice.

In research on clinical teaching effectiveness, students have consistently reported that the teacher must be knowledgeable about the clinical practice area, able to share that knowledge and expertise with them as they learn to care for patients, and current in the specialty (Beitz & Wieland, 2005; Benor & Leviyof, 1997; Gignac-Caille & Oermann, 2001; Tang, Chou, & Chiang, 2005). Being knowledgeable about the clinical practice area includes

- understanding concepts and theories that relate to the care of patients in the clinical setting;

- assisting students to *use* those concepts and theories to better understand their patients' health problems and care;

- being up-to-date on research in nursing and health care that relates to the clinical area, nursing interventions and how they might be used in the care of patients with whom students are working, evidence-based practice, and new technologies;

- using this clinical knowledge to help students arrive at sound decisions about patient care.

In a study by Tang and colleagues (2005), having "sufficient professional knowledge" was one of the three highest ranked clinical teacher behaviors. In another study, Wolf and associates (2004) analyzed student evaluations of faculty performance and found that strengths of the teacher included patterns such as being knowledgeable, creating a positive learning environment, being professional and supportive of students, and displaying scholarly attributes.

Clinical Competence

Teachers cannot guide student learning in clinical practice without being competent themselves. Clinical competence is an important characteristic of effective clinical teaching in nursing (Benor & Leviyof, 1997; Cahill, 1997; Gignac-Caille & Oermann, 2001; Tang, Chou, & Chiang, 2005). In a study by Gignac-Caille and Oermann (2001), 292 students in various levels of their associate degree nursing programs identified "demonstrates clinical skills and judgment" as the most important characteristic of effective clinical instructors. The best teachers are experts in their clinical specialty, have maintained their clinical skills, can demonstrate nursing care in a real situation, and can guide students in developing essential clinical competencies.

This quality of teaching may be problematic for faculty who teach predominantly in the classroom or change practice settings frequently and do not keep current in their clinical specialty. In some schools of nursing, clinical faculty are required to maintain a clinical practice certification, which encourages continued competency. For programs without such a requirement, it is up to the teacher to maintain clinical expertise and skills.

Skill in Clinical Teaching

Skill in clinical teaching includes the ability of the teacher to assess learning needs, plan instruction that meets those needs and fosters achievement of the outcomes of the clinical course, guide students in developing their clinical competencies, and evaluate learning fairly. These teaching skills are described more specifically in Table 4.1.

The clinical teacher needs to know *how to teach*. While this skill seems obvious, in some settings clinical teachers, preceptors, and others working with students are not educationally prepared for their roles. They have limited knowledge about how to guide students' learning in the clinical setting and evaluate their performance (Oermann, 2004). Being an expert clinician is not enough—the teacher must know how to teach.

In a study by Berg and Lindseth (2004), the instructional skills of the teacher were ranked second highest when students (n = 171) were asked to describe

TABLE 4.1   Clinical Teaching Skills

- Assess of learning needs of students, recognizing and accepting differences
- Plans or assignments that help in the transfer of learning to clinical practice, meet learning needs, and promote acquisition of knowledge and development of competencies
- Communicates clearly to students the outcomes of learning and expectations of students in clinical practice
- Considers student goals and needs in planning clinical activities
- Structures clinical assignments and activities in clinical practice so they build on one another
- Explains clearly concepts and theories applicable to patient care
- Demonstrates effectively clinical skills, procedures, and use of technology
- Provides opportunities for practice of clinical skills, procedures, and technology and recognizes of differences among students in the amount of practice needed
- Is well-prepared for clinical teaching
- Develops clinical teaching strategies that encourage students to problem solve, arrive at clinical decisions, and think critically in a clinical situation
- Asks higher-level questions that assist students in thinking through complex clinical situations and cases requiring critical thinking
- Encourages students through teaching and evaluation to think independently and beyond accepted practices and to try out new interventions
- Plans varied clinical teaching strategies and learning activities to stimulate student interest and meet individual needs of students
- Guides learning and students' use of resources for learning
- Available to students in clinical practice when they need assistance
- Models professional role behaviors for students
- Provides specific, timely, and useful feedback on student progress
- Shares observations of clinical performance with students
- Encourages students to evaluate their own performance
- Corrects mistakes without belittling students
- Is fair in evaluation

characteristics of an effective teacher in nursing. When those same students were asked about ineffective teachers, lack of teaching skill was ranked highest.

The best clinical teachers

- assess each student's learning needs;
- plan patient assignments and other clinical activities that are individualized, reflect the competencies to be developed, and are appropriate to the student's current level of knowledge and skill;

- promote transfer of learning to the clinical setting by asking questions and planning teaching strategies that help students think about how theory relates to their patients;

- ask higher level questions that encourage critical thinking and are consistent with the student's level of understanding;

- give clear explanations and directions;

- effectively demonstrate procedures and clinical skills;

- serve as a role model for students;

- provide time for students to develop their clinical competencies before grading their performance;

- create a climate that is supportive of students as they develop their clinical skills and in which students are comfortable to ask questions when unsure;

- provide immediate and honest feedback, combined with suggestions as to how students can improve their performance.

Skills in evaluating clinical performance—both formatively, for feedback, and summatively, at the end of a period of time in the clinical course—are critical for effective teaching. Research has shown that effective teachers are fair in their evaluations of students, correct student errors without belittling students and diminishing their self-confidence, and give prompt feedback that promotes further learning and development.

Interpersonal Relationships With Students

The ability of the clinical teacher to interact with students, both on a one-to-one basis and as a clinical group, is another important teacher behavior. Qualities of an effective teacher in this area are showing confidence in students, respecting them, being honest and direct, supporting students and demonstrating caring behaviors, being approachable, and encouraging students to ask questions and seek guidance when needed. In Gignac-Caille and Oermann's (2001) study of effective clinical teaching, the 10 most important characteristics identified by faculty were composed of behaviors from the subscales of interpersonal relationships and teaching skills. Considering the demands on students as they learn to care for patients, students need to view the teacher as someone who supports them in their learning.

Manias and Aitken (2005) emphasized the important role of the clinical teacher in providing this support to nursing students.

Personal Characteristics of Clinical Teacher

Personal attributes of the teacher also influence teaching effectiveness. These attributes include enthusiasm, a sense of humor, willingness to admit limitations and mistakes honestly, patience, and flexibility when working with students in the clinical setting, among others (Berg & Lindseth, 2004; Gignac-Caille & Oermann, 2001; Tang, Chou, & Chiang, 2005). Students often describe effective teachers as ones who are friendly and provide an opportunity for them to share feelings and concerns about patients. Tang and colleagues (2005) found that most of the differences between effective and ineffective teachers related to the interpersonal relationships and personality characteristics categories. In a study by Berg and Lindseth (2004), personality was the most frequently mentioned quality of an effective teacher with comments such as "easy to get along with."

Three other personal qualities important in teaching in any setting are integrity, perseverance, and courage (Glassick, Huber, & Maeroff, 1997). While these characteristics were originally used to describe the teacher as a scholar, they are just as important in carrying out the clinical teaching role. Integrity implies truthfulness with students and fairness in dealing with them in the process of learning and in clinical evaluation. The teacher develops an atmosphere of trust for students to engage in open discussions, examine alternatives, and discuss conflicting opinions with the faculty. Fairness "involves the presentation of one's own interpretations and conclusions in ways that keep open an examination of alternatives" (Glassick et al., 1997, p. 64).

In clinical teaching, faculty members need to persevere in their efforts to improve their teaching competencies. They should be willing to reflect on their teaching and evaluation practices and consider better ways of designing clinical activities and guiding students in their learning. Good teachers, like good scholars, strive to perfect their teaching skills over time and avoid stagnation in their teaching approaches.

Glassick et al. (1997) described courage as risking disapproval, having the will to take on difficult or unpopular ideas, transcending traditional views, and imagining new questions and approaches (p. 65). Courage enables the teacher to suggest new approaches to organizing the clinical practicum, propose different methods for clinical instruction, question established clinical evaluation practices, and ask if there are better ways of teaching students and judging their clinical performance.

STRESSES OF STUDENTS IN CLINICAL PRACTICE

Students

Clinical practice is inherently stressful. In the clinical setting, students face uncertainties and unique situations that they may not have encountered in their prior learning. For some students, it is stressful to practice providing care because they are unsure about approaches and interventions to use. Students fear making a mistake that would harm the patient, and in pediatric nursing courses they often worry about administering medications and the possibility of making medication errors (Oermann & Lukomski, 2001). Interacting with the teacher, other health care providers, the patient, and family members also may contribute to the stress that students experience in clinical practice.

Other stresses, from the students' perspective, relate to the changing nature of patient conditions, a lack of knowledge and skill to provide care to patients, unfamiliarity in the clinical setting, working with difficult patients, developing technological skills, and clinical evaluation and being observed by the teacher (Oermann, 1998a; Oermann & Lukomski, 2001; Oermann & Moffitt-Wolf, 1997; Oermann & Sperling, 1999; Shipton, 2002). Students in clinical courses in baccalaureate nursing programs also indicate that the paperwork often required for the clinical practicum is an added source of stress for them (Oermann, 1998a).

The stress that students experience in clinical practice is not consistent across clinical courses and settings. In a number of studies, stress was highest for students enrolled in pediatric nursing clinical courses and lowest for foundations courses (Oermann & Lukomski, 2001; Oermann & Sperling, 1999; Oermann & Standfest, 1997). Students also may experience greater stress in clinical practice at different points in the nursing curriculum. Oermann (1998a) found, for instance, that the stress experienced by students in clinical practice in both associate degree (ADN) and bachelor of science (BSN) programs increased as they progressed through the program; the semester prior to graduation was the most stressful time in terms of clinical practice for both groups of students. Preceptorships may also be highly stressful for students as both preceptor and student strive to accommodate one another in a new professional relationship (Yonge, Myrick, & Haase, 2002).

Many of these studies found that the clinical teacher and behaviors of the teacher created the most stress for students. This finding reinforces the need for the faculty to develop supportive and trusting relationships with students in the clinical setting and to be aware of the stressful nature of clinical learning activities. A climate that supports the process of learning in clinical practice depends on a caring relationship between teacher and student rather than an adversarial one. Cook (2005) found that when teachers convey inviting messages—such as showing respect for students, expressing pleasure with the clinical group, and being friendly, among others—students reported less anxiety. Learning in clinical practice occurs in public under the watchful eye of the teacher, the patient, and others in the setting. By keeping the nature of clinical learning in mind and using supportive and inviting behaviors when interacting with students, the teacher can reduce some of the stress that students naturally feel in clinical practice.

Sprengel and Job (2004) developed a peer mentoring program to reduce the stress of students during their initial hospital clinical experience. Both the beginning students who were mentored and the sophomore students who served as their peer mentors described benefits of this program including reducing stress in the clinical environment.

STRESSFUL NATURE OF CLINICAL TEACHING

Teachers

Clinical teaching can be stressful for the teacher. First, it is time consuming. A three-credit theory or online course usually requires 3 hours per week of instruction, 1 clock hour for each credit hour, not including preparation time. However, a three-credit clinical course may require 6 to 9 hours of clinical teaching a week, 2 to 3 clinical practice hours per credit hour, and even more in some nursing education programs. This time commitment for clinical teaching may create stress for faculty members who are also involved in research, scholarship, and faculty practice. In many nursing education programs, faculty members are responsible for writing grants, conducting research, writing for publication, serving on committees, providing community service, and maintaining a clinical practice. These multiple roles are demanding and could lead to role conflict and job dissatisfaction (Gormley, 2003).

In addition to demands associated with the multiple roles of a nursing faculty member, other aspects of clinical teaching may be stressful. These include

- coping with job expectations associated with clinical teaching;
- feeling physically and emotionally drained at the end of a clinical teaching day;
- job demands that interfere with activities of personal importance;
- heavy workload;
- pressure to maintain clinical competence or a clinical practice without time to do so;

- feeling unable to satisfy the demands of work-related constituencies (students, clinical agency personnel, patients, and others);

- teaching inadequately prepared students (Oermann, 1998b).

Novice faculty members and teachers new to a nursing education program should find a mentor in the school who can provide advice and suggestions for coping with the stresses associated with clinical teaching and managing their varied faculty roles. Bellack (2003) recommended that every new faculty member seek early and ongoing support from his or her department chair, director, or other mentor and learn what it takes to be successful in that program. These individuals can be good sources of guidance on how to balance clinical teaching with other faculty roles. Faculty on the tenure track may need release time from clinical teaching responsibilities to work on research and scholarship; changes in workload should be negotiated early in one's career to allow adequate time for scholarly activities.

SOCIALIZATION OF STUDENTS

Socialization is the process through which students acquire the knowledge, skills, and values for professional practice. Although there are various theoretical perspectives of professional socialization, consistent among them is the notion that through this process the person acquires necessary behaviors to function in a particular role. Socialization is frequently viewed within the perspective of role theory. In this process, by working with someone in the role, the student gains essential knowledge, behaviors, and values for carrying out the role.

Clinical education provides the avenue for acquiring the knowledge and behaviors for practice in a particular role, whether it is a beginning professional nurse or a new role such as advanced practice nurse. This process requires learning about the role, as the initial step, and observing and working with nurses in that role, as the second step. The teacher guides the student in learning about the role of the nurse and role behaviors, and models important values and attributes of the professional in that role. If there is a caring relationship between the teacher and student with honest and open communication, then students can more easily internalize the behaviors and values they are learning about into their own practice (Hentz, 2005). Socialization comes from an integration of clinical and other experiences, not only from the guidance of the teacher. The experiences of students with preceptors, other nurses, and other health care providers contribute to this socialization process.

MODELS OF CLINICAL TEACHING

There are different models of clinical teaching: traditional, in which the teacher is directly responsible for guiding students in the clinical setting; preceptor; and partnership. In the preceptor and partnership models, preceptors, advanced practice nurses, and others in the clinical setting provide the clinical instruction with a faculty member responsible for overall planning, coordinating the experience, grading clinical practice, and assuming other course-related responsibilities.

Traditional Model

In the traditional model of clinical teaching, the educator provides the instruction and evaluation for a small group of nursing students and is on-site during the clinical experience. A benefit of this model is the opportunity to assist students in using the concepts and theories learned in class, through online instruction, in readings, and through other learning activities in patient care. The teacher can select clinical activities that best meet the students' needs and are consistent with course goals and objectives. Since the clinical teacher is involved to varying degrees with the nursing curriculum overall, the clinical activities may be more carefully selected to reflect the concepts and theories that students are learning in the course than when preceptor or partners provide the instruction. In addition, the faculty member may be more committed to implementing the philosophy of the nursing program than preceptors or clinicians hired only for clinical teaching, often on a short-term basis.

Disadvantages, though, are the large number of students for whom faculty members may be responsible; not being accessible to students when needed because of demands of other students in the group; teaching procedures, clinical skills, and use of technologies for which the faculty member may lack expertise; and the time commitment of providing on-site clinical instruction for faculty members with multiple other roles. Faculty members who are part-time or adjunct may not be sufficiently familiar with the philosophy of the program, overall curriculum, clinical competencies developed prior to and following the course in which they are teaching, and other program characteristics, which may affect their planning of clinical activities for students and their expectations of students in the course. It is critical for the full-time faculty to prepare and orient part-time and adjunct faculty members involved in clinical teaching so they are not only aware of their role and responsibilities but also understand how their course relates to the overall nursing curriculum.

Another disadvantage of the traditional model of clinical teaching is that often the educator and students are not part of the health care system in which students have clinical practice. They are outsiders to the clinical setting and may not understand the system of care in that setting and its culture. As such, faculty members must work closely with the managers and clinical nursing staff to ensure an effective clinical experience for students. It is up to the faculty member to develop a working relationship with the staff, which is essential to create an environment for learning and to take advantage of experiences available in the setting. In the traditional model of clinical teaching, faculty who are not also practicing in the clinical setting often invest extensive time in developing and maintaining these relationships.

The relationships that nursing faculty members develop in the clinical setting are not only with nursing staff but also involve other health care providers, particularly when the goals of clinical education are interdisciplinary in nature. With overlapping roles and responsibilities of health care providers and emphasis on interdisciplinary care, nursing students need clinical learning activities in which they examine their own role in relationship to other providers and collaborate with other health professionals (Gilbert, 2005; Mayne & Glascoff, 2002; Rodehorst, Wilhelm, & Jensen, 2005). These activities can be integrated within a nursing course, or nursing students can participate in courses with other health professional students (White, Zapka, Coghlin-Strom, Alexander, & Bauer-Wu, 2004).

Preceptor Model

In the preceptor model of clinical teaching, an expert nurse in the clinical setting works with the student on a one-to-one basis in the clinical setting. Preceptors are staff nurses and other nurses employed by the clinical agency who in addition to their ongoing patient care responsibilities provide on-site clinical instruction for the assigned students. In addition to one-to-one teaching, the preceptor guides and supports the learner and serves as a role model. Preceptorships provide a vehicle for transitioning students into professional practice, socializing them into their professional role, and bridging the juncture between the classroom and clinical setting (Myrick & Yonge, 2003, p. 93).

In the preceptor model of clinical instruction, the faculty member from the nursing program serves as the course coordinator, liaison between the nursing education program and clinical setting, and resource person for the preceptor. The faculty member, however, is typically not on-site during the clinical practicum. The preceptor model involves sharing clinical teaching responsibilities between nursing program faculty and expert clinicians from the practice setting. Guidelines for setting up a preceptorship are described in Chapter 14.

One strength of the preceptor model is the consistent one-to-one relationship of the student and preceptor, providing an opportunity for the student to work closely with a role model. This close relationship promotes socialization and enables students to gain an understanding of how to function in the role for which they are being prepared. Precepted learning activities are an appropriate way to deal with concerns that students are not adequately prepared to meet employer expectations at the time of graduation (Myrick & Yonge, 2003). Other advantages of preceptorships are that students are able to work closely with a clinical expert in the field, develop self-confidence, improve their critical thinking and decision-making skills, and learn new clinical skills under the guidance of the preceptor.

Potential disadvantages of the preceptor model are lack of integration of theory, research, and practice; lack of flexibility in reassigning students to other preceptors if needed; and time and other demands made on the preceptors. Although preceptors should be prepared educationally for this role, some preceptors may lack clinical teaching skills.

The preceptor model is commonly used at upper levels of the prelicensure curriculum, often in the final clinical course; for graduate nursing students; and in distance education courses. However, preceptors can also be used with beginning nursing students, providing an opportunity for them to develop their clinical knowledge and skills guided by an expert in the role and gain a realistic view of clinical practice. In distance education courses, when students do not live locally, clinical settings can be established close to the students' homes with preceptors providing the clinical instruction; guidelines for choosing, orienting, and using preceptors in a distance education program are described in Chapter 10.

Nursing education programs have different systems in place for choosing preceptors. Myrick and Yonge (2003) recommend that preceptors in local health care settings be chosen collaboratively by the nurse manager on the unit and the faculty member responsible for the practicum. For distance education courses, students can suggest their own preceptors who are then reviewed by the nursing program faculty; this process is discussed in Chapter 10. In other programs national networking provides a pool of preceptors in distant areas (Baldwin & Burns, 2004). Once chosen, preceptors must be prepared for their teaching role and oriented thoroughly to the course, its outcomes, and the roles of student, preceptor, faculty, and others involved in the experience. This orientation should emphasize the evaluation process and how to provide both positive and negative feedback to learners (Mamchur & Myrick, 2003).

Partnership Model

There are varied types of partnerships in nursing education. Many of these are the result of nursing program faculties and administrators searching for ways to increase student enrollment and cope with budgetary constraints, a nursing faculty shortage, and not enough clinical sites, combined with health care agencies experiencing a nursing shortage (American Association of Colleges of Nursing [AACN], 2002; Oermann, 2004). In partnerships, nursing education programs collaborate with clinical agencies to respond to these issues as well as to meet the health care needs of the community.

Partnerships vary widely. In some programs the partnership model is a collaborative relationship between a clinical agency and nursing program that involves sharing an advanced practice nurse (APN) and academic faculty member. The APN teaches students in the clinical setting, with the faculty member serving as course coordinator, and the faculty member, in turn, contributes to the clinical agency, for example, by conducting research and serving as a consultant. Expertise and services are shared between the partners. In this type of partnership, the APN may work with a graduate nursing student on an individualized basis or may teach a group of prelicensure students, as in the traditional clinical teaching model. At both the undergraduate and graduate levels, the faculty member works closely with the APN to ensure the selection of relevant clinical activities for students.

Another example of a partnership for clinical teaching is the clinical partner model. In this model, a faculty member teaches two groups of students, as in the traditional model, but is partnered with two clinical adjunct instructors from the clinical setting. Each of the adjunct instructors is assigned to one of these clinical groups (Campbell & Dudley, 2005). This model provides a way of doubling the capacity of the nursing faculty and gives the students an opportunity to be mentored and taught by expert clinicians practicing in that setting.

Other partnerships are community based, linking education, practice, and research (Plowfield, Wheeler, & Raymond, 2005; Shellenbarger, 2003; Tagliareni & Speakman, 2003). Falk-Rafael, Ward-Griffin, Laforet-Fliesser, and Beynon (2004) described their community-based model, which includes partnerships between the school of nursing and several health departments, community health centers, and many community groups. Other levels of partnerships are also apparent, for example, partnerships among faculty, agency advisors, and students; students partnering with the community; and students partnering with each other (Falk-Rafael et al., 2004).

Other nursing education programs have instituted partnerships to meet specific curriculum goals. For example, one school initiated partnerships with four area health care agencies employing licensed practical nurses (LPNs) to facilitate their obtaining a BSN. The agencies supported students with full or partial tuition reimbursement and work schedules that accommodated their classes. The program also included role transition seminars, faculty members who served as mentors to the LPN students, and preceptors who served as clinical mentors and "professional partners," among other components (Ramsey, Merriman, Blowers, Grooms, & Sullivan, 2004).

Selecting a Clinical Teaching Model

There is no one model that meets the need of every nursing program, clinical course, or group of students. The teacher should select a model considering these factors

- educational philosophy of the nursing program;

- philosophy of the faculty about clinical teaching;

- goals and intended outcomes of the clinical course and activities;

- level of nursing student;

- type of clinical setting;

- availability of preceptors, expert nurses, and other people in the practice setting to provide clinical instruction;

- willingness of clinical agency personnel and partners to participate in teaching students and in other educational activities.

SUMMARY

Teaching in the clinical setting requires a faculty member who is knowledgeable, is clinically competent, knows how to teach, relates effectively to students, and is enthusiastic about clinical teaching. The research in nursing education over the years has substantiated that these qualities are important in clinical teaching. Students describe an effective clinical teacher as one who displays these behaviors; they describe an ineffective teacher as one who lacks these qualities.

Clinical practice is inherently stressful for students. While some clinical courses may be more stressful than others, students have identified dimensions of clinical learning that are often anxiety producing, such as fear of making a mistake that would harm the patient; interacting with the patient, the teacher, and other health care providers; the changing nature of patient conditions; a lack of knowledge and skill to practice giving care to patients; and working with difficult patients, among others. In some research, students have reported that the teacher is a source of added stress for them. These findings highlight the need for faculty members to develop supportive and trusting relationships with students in the clinical setting and to be aware of the stressful nature of this learning experience. A climate that supports the process of learning in clinical practice depends on a caring relationship between teacher and student rather than an adversarial one.

Serving as a role model for students, or selecting clinicians who will model important professional behaviors and the role for which the student is preparing, is also important in clinical teaching. Working with a role model in clinical practice facilitates the student's own socialization into the professional role, either as a beginning nurse or when preparing for a new role such as an APN.

The teacher also chooses a model for clinical teaching: traditional, preceptor, or partnership. In the traditional model of clinical teaching, the instruction and evaluation of a group of students are carried out by a faculty member who is on-site during the clinical experience. A benefit of this model is the opportunity to assist students in applying concepts to the care of patients. The teacher can plan clinical learning activities that best meet the students' needs and are consistent with course goals and objectives.

In the preceptor model of clinical teaching, an expert nurse (the preceptor) in the clinical setting works with the student on a one to one basis. In addition to his or her ongoing patient care responsibilities, the preceptor provides on-site clinical instruction for the assigned student. He or she also guides and supports the learner and serves as a role model. The faculty member is typically not on-site during the clinical experience but has important responsibilities for the course such as serving as course coordinator, providing the classroom instruction, serving as liaison between the nursing education program and clinical setting, and being a resource person for the preceptor.

Partnerships were also described in this chapter. The partnership model varies with the academic institution but generally is a collaborative relationship between the nursing education program and a clinical agency or among varied agencies in the community. In some partnerships an APN teaches students in the clinical setting, with the faculty member contributing in other ways to the clinical agency. Partnerships emphasize collaboration among partners to meet the needs of the partners and community as a whole.

The teacher chooses a model after considering the educational philosophy of the nursing education program and faculty, goals of the clinical course, characteristics of the clinical setting, availability and willingness of agencies to partner with the program, and characteristics of the students, among other factors. In all of the models of clinical teaching, the teacher, regardless of whether that person is from the nursing education program or clinical setting, is critical to creating a climate for learning, supporting students as they gain new knowledge and clinical skills, and serving as a role model for them.

REFERENCES

American Association of Colleges of Nursing. (2002, October). Using strategic partnerships to expand nursing education programs. *AACN Issue Bulletin*. Retrieved January 17, 2006, from http://www.aacn.nche.edu/Publications/issues/Oct02.htm

Baldwin, K. M., & Burns, P. G. (2004). Development and implementation of an online CNS program. *Clinical Nurse Specialist, 18*, 248–254.

Beitz, J. M., & Wieland, D. (2005). Analyzing the teaching effectiveness of clinical nursing faculty of full- and part-time generic BSN, LPN-BSN, and RN-BSN nursing students. *Journal of Professional Nursing, 21*, 32–45.

Bellack, J. P. (2003). Advice for new (and seasoned) faculty. *Journal of Nursing Education, 42*, 383–384.

Benor, D. E., & Leviyof, I. (1997). The development of students' perceptions of effective teaching: The ideal, best, and poorest clinical teacher in nursing. *Journal of Nursing Education, 36*, 206–211.

Berg, C. L., & Lindseth, G. (2004). Research brief. Students' perspectives of effective and ineffective nursing instructors. *Journal of Nursing Education, 43*, 565–568.

Cahill, H. A. (1997). What should nurse teachers be doing? A preliminary study. *Journal of Advanced Nursing, 26*, 146–153.

Campbell, S. E., & Dudley, K. (2005). Clinical partner model: Benefits for education and service. *Nurse Educator, 30*, 271–274.

Cook, L. J. (2005). Inviting teaching behaviors of clinical faculty and nursing students' anxiety. *Journal of Nursing Education, 44*, 156–161.

Falk-Rafael, A. R., Ward-Griffin, C., Laforet-Fliesser, Y., & Beynon, C. (2004). Teaching nursing students to promote the health of communities: A partnership approach. *Nurse Educator, 29*, 63–67.

Gignac-Caille, A. M., & Oermann, M. H. (2001). Student and faculty perceptions of effective clinical instructors in ADN programs. *Journal of Nursing Education, 40*, 347–353.

Gilbert, J. H. V. (2005). Interprofessional education for collaborative, patient-centred practice. *Canadian Journal of Nursing Leadership, 18*, 32–36, 38.

Glassick, C. E., Huber, M. T., & Maeroff, G. I. (1997). *Scholarship assessed.* San Francisco: Jossey-Bass.

Gormley, D. K. (2003). Factors affecting job satisfaction in nurse faculty: A meta-analysis. *Journal of Nursing Education, 42*, 174–178.

Hentz, P. B. (2005). Education and socialization to the professional nursing role. In K. Masters (Ed.), *Role development in professional nursing practice* (pp. 99–109). Sudbury, MA: Jones and Bartlett.

Mamchur, C., & Myrick, F. (2003). Preceptorship and interpersonal conflict: A multidisciplinary study. *Journal of Advanced Nursing, 43*, 188–196.

Manias, E., & Aitken, R. (2005). Clinical teachers in specialty practice settings: Perceptions of their role within postgraduate nursing programs. *Learning in Health and Social Care, 4*, 67–77.

Mayne, L., & Glascoff, M. (2002). Service learning: Preparing a healthcare workforce for the next century. *Nurse Educator, 27*, 191–194.

Myrick, F., & Yonge, O. (2003). Preceptorship: A quintessential component of nursing education. In M. H. Oermann & K. T. Heinrich (Eds.), *Annual review of nursing education* (Vol. 1, pp. 91–107). New York: Springer Publishing.

Oermann, M. H. (1998a). Differences in clinical experiences of ADN and BSN students. *Journal of Nursing Education, 37*, 197–201.

Oermann, M. H. (1998b). Work-related stresses of clinical nursing faculty. *Journal of Nursing Education, 37*, 302–304.

Oermann, M. H. (2004). Reflections on undergraduate nursing education: A look to the future. *International Journal of Nursing Education Scholarship, 1*(1), 1–15. Retrieved from http://www.bepress.com/ijnes/vol1/iss1/art5

Oermann, M. H., & Lukomski, A. P. (2001). Experiences of students in pediatric nursing clinical courses. *Journal of the Society of Pediatric Nurses, 9*, 65–72.

Oermann, M. H., & Moffitt-Wolf, A. (1997). Graduate nurses' perceptions of clinical practice. *Journal of Continuing Education in Nursing, 28*, 20–25.

Oermann, M. H., & Sperling, S. L. (1999). Stress and challenge of psychiatric nursing clinical experiences. *Archives of Psychiatric Nursing, XIII*(2), 74–79.

Oermann, M. H., & Standfest, K. M. (1997). Differences in stress and challenge in clinical practice among ADN and BSN students in varying clinical courses. *Journal of Nursing Education, 36*, 228–233.

Plowfield, L. A., Wheeler, E. C., & Raymond, J. E. (2005). Time, tact, talent, and trust: Essential ingredients of effective academic-community partnerships. *Nursing Education Perspectives, 26*, 217–220.

Ramsey, P., Merriman, C., Blowers, S., Grooms, J., & Sullivan, K. (2004). Community partnerships for an LPN to BSN career mobility project. *Nurse Educator, 29*, 31–35.

Rodehorst, T. K., Wilhelm, S. L., & Jensen L. (2005). Use of interdisciplinary simulation to understand perceptions of team members' roles. *Journal of Professional Nursing, 21*, 159–166.

Shellenbarger, T. (2003). Professional-community partnerships: Successful collaboration. In M. H. Oermann & K. T. Heinrich (Eds.), *Annual review of nursing education* (Vol. 1, pp. 43–58). New York: Springer Publishing.

Shipton, S. P. (2002). The process of seeking stress-care: Coping as experienced by senior baccalaureate nursing students in response to appraised clinical stress. *Journal of Nursing Education, 41*, 243–256.

Sprengel, A. D., & Job, L. (2004). Reducing student anxiety by using clinical peer mentoring with beginning nursing students. *Nurse Educator, 29*, 246–250.

Tagliareni, M. E., & Speakman, E. (2003). Community-based curricula at ADN level: A service-learning model. In M. H. Oermann & K. T. Heinrich (Eds.), *Annual review of nursing education* (Vol. 1, pp. 27–41). New York: Springer Publishing.

Tang, F., Chou, S., & Chiang, H. (2005). Students' perceptions of effective and ineffective clinical instructors. *Journal of Nursing Education, 44*, 187–192.

White, M. J., Zapka, J. G., Coghlin-Strom, J., Alexander, M. K., & Bauer-Wu, S. (2004). Interdisciplinary collaboration for health professional education in cancer control. *Journal of Cancer Education, 19*, 37–44.

Wolf, Z. R., Bender, P. J., Beitz, J. M., Wieland, D. M., & Vito, K. O. (2004). Strengths and weaknesses of faculty teaching performance reported by undergraduate and graduate nursing students: A descriptive study. *Journal of Professional Nursing, 20*, 118–128.

Yonge, O., Myrick, F., & Haase, M. (2002). Student nurse stress in the preceptorship experience. *Nurse Educator, 27*, 84–88.

Chapter 5

Process of Clinical Teaching

Clinical teaching is a complex interaction of student and teacher within the context of the environment in which it occurs. Characteristics of the teacher and learner; the clinical environment and nature of practice within that environment; patients, families, and others for whom students are caring; agency personnel and other health care providers; and the inherent nature of clinical practice with its uncertainties all influence the teaching process. With many clinical activities, the teacher and student are outsiders to the clinical setting and are perceived as guests; this perception, too, influences clinical teaching and learning.

The process of clinical teaching is described in this chapter, but the reader should be cognizant that this process is not prescriptive. Instead, it provides a framework for the teacher to use in planning clinical activities appropriate for the learning outcomes and students, guiding students in the practice setting, and evaluating clinical performance. A framework assists faculty in creating an environment and opportunities for students to learn; the outcomes of those experiences, however, may vary considerably among students because of the many factors that influence the learning process. A framework for clinical teaching guides the teacher in decision making about clinical teaching but in no way guarantees that certain learning outcomes will occur for every student.

TEACHING AND LEARNING

Teaching is a complex process intended to facilitate learning. While the goal of teaching is to lead students in discovering knowledge for themselves, the teacher encourages this discovery through deliberate teaching actions that lead in that direction. Self-discovery does not imply a lack of structure; instead, the teacher provides structure and learning activities for self-discovery by the student.

Teaching is a series of deliberate actions on the part of the teacher to guide students in their learning. It involves a sharing and mutual experience on the part of both teacher and student and is carried out in an environment of support and trust. Teaching is not telling, it is not dispensing information, and it is not merely demonstrating skills. Instead, teaching is *involving* the student as an active participant in this learning. The teacher is a resource person with information to share for the purpose of facilitating learning and acquisition of new knowledge and skills.

Learning is a process through which people change as a result of their experiences. Some people view learning as an overt and a measurable change in behavior resulting from an experience; however, this view negates a change in perception and insight as learning. In the clinical setting, new insights, ideas, and perspectives may be just as critical to the student's learning and development as overt and measurable behaviors. Learning, therefore, may be a change in observable behavior or performance, or it may reflect a new perception and insight not manifested by an overt change in behavior.

The teaching–learning process is a complex interaction of these processes. The teacher is a facilitator of learning, and the student is an active participant. The need for students to be actively involved in their learning is critical in the teaching–learning process, particularly in the clinical setting. When students are actively involved in their learning and perceive a positive teacher–student relationship, they can be honest about their learning needs and how faculty can help them in developing their clinical competencies.

Active learning also fosters critical thinking because students can explore alternate perspectives and different decisions that could be made in a clinical situation (Oermann, 1998, 2004). With active learning, students improve problem-solving skills and learn how to use knowledge in clinical practice (Richardson & Trudeau, 2003). They can think about and discuss with others how concepts and theories are used to solve clinical problems. By being actively involved in their learning, students can reflect on their clinical experience and put their thoughts into words, which leads to new knowledge and deeper learning (Murphy, 2005).

Although teaching and learning are interrelated processes, each may occur without the other. Significant learning may result from the student's clinical activities without any teacher involvement. Similarly, the teacher's carefully planned assignments and activities for students may not lead to any new learning or development of competencies. The goal of clinical instruction is to create the *environment and activities for learning*, recognizing that each student will gain different insights and outcomes from them.

PROCESS OF CLINICAL TEACHING: FIVE COMPONENTS

The process of clinical teaching includes five steps:

1. Identifying the outcomes for learning
2. Assessing learning needs
3. Planning clinical learning activities
4. Guiding learners in clinical practice
5. Evaluating clinical learning and performance.

The process of clinical teaching is not linear; instead, each component influences others. For example, clinical evaluation provides data on further learning needs of students that, in turn, suggest new learning activities. Similarly, as the teacher works with students, observations of performance may alter the assessment and suggest different learning activities.

Identifying Outcomes for Learning

The first step in clinical teaching is to identify the goals and outcomes of the clinical experience. These intended learning goals and outcomes suggest areas for assessment, provide guidelines for teaching, and are the basis for evaluating learning. Faculties identify these outcomes in different ways. In some nursing programs, the outcomes of learning are stated as objectives to be achieved by students in the clinical course. In other programs they are expressed in the form of clinical competencies to be demonstrated at the end of the course or for specific clinical activities. The competencies may indicate the knowledge that students should gain in the clinical practicum, values that should be demonstrated when providing care and working with staff, and specific psychomotor and technological skills in which students need to be proficient.

Clinical competencies often address eight areas of learning. These general areas are listed here with examples of competencies in each area.

1. Knowledge, concepts, and theories used in clinical practice
    *   Relates research on pain management interventions to care of patients in acute pain.
    *   Applies multicultural concepts of care to the community as client.
2. Assessment, diagnosis, plan, interventions, and evaluation of outcomes
    *   Collects data that are developmentally and age appropriate for healthy and ill children.

- Considers multiple nursing interventions, weighing the consequences of each.

3. Psychomotor and technological skills and other types of interventions
    - Competently provides wound care.
    - Demonstrates skill in conducting a physical examination.

4. Values related to care of patients, families, and communities and other dimensions of health care
    - Recognizes personal values that might conflict with professional nursing values.
    - Accepts cultural, ethnic, and other differences of patients and communities.

5. Communication skills, ability to develop interpersonal relationships, and skill in collaboration with others
    - Collaborates with other health care providers in interdisciplinary care of children with disabilities.
    - Communicates effectively with patients, families, staff, and others in the health care setting.

6. Management of care, leadership abilities, and role behaviors
    - Manages care effectively for a small group of patients.
    - Demonstrates the role and behaviors of a nurse as leader.

7. Accountability and responsibility of the learner
    - Accepts responsibility for own actions and decisions.
    - Provides safe nursing care.

8. Self-development and continued learning
    - Identifies own learning needs in clinical practice.
    - Seeks learning opportunities to develop clinical competencies.

In some clinical courses students need to demonstrate learning and performance in all of these areas as well as in others specific to the clinical specialty or setting. Other courses may focus on only a few of these areas of learning. Clinical competencies may be stated broadly similar to most of the preceding examples, or they can be more specific, such as, "administer intravenous injection of medications." In any clinical course the competencies should be achievable by students considering their prior knowledge, skills, and experiences; clinical learning opportunities available in the setting; and time allotted for clinical practice.

The clinical competencies should be communicated clearly to students, in written form, and understood by them. Similarly, the teacher has an important responsibility in *discussing* these outcomes and related clinical activities with agency personnel, not *telling* them. Agency personnel need input into decisions about the clinical activities and their match with the goals, philosophy, and care delivery system of the clinical setting. With this input, the teacher may need to alter intended clinical activities and plan simulations and other types of learning opportunities for students.

Students also should have input into the clinical competencies; there may be some already achieved by students and others to be added to meet their individual learning needs and goals. There should be some flexibility in the clinical course as long as students demonstrate the competencies and achieve the essential knowledge and skills for progressing through the nursing program.

Assessing Learning Needs

Teaching begins at the level of the learner. The teacher's goal, therefore, is to assess the student's present level of knowledge and skill and other characteristics that may influence achieving the outcomes of the clinical practicum. The first area of assessment involves collecting data on whether the student has the prerequisite knowledge and skills for the clinical situation at hand and for completing the learning activities. For instance, if the learning activities focus on interventions for health promotion, students first need some understanding of health and behaviors for promoting health. Changing a sterile dressing requires an understanding of principles of asepsis. The teacher's role in assessment of the learner is important so that students engage in learning activities that build on their present knowledge and skills. When students lack the prerequisites, then the instruction can help students learn this information and more efficiently move students forward in their learning.

Not every student will enter the clinical course with the same prerequisite knowledge and skills, depending on past learning and clinical experiences. The teacher, therefore, should not expect the same entry competencies for all students. Assessment reveals the point at which the instruction should begin and does not imply poor performance for students, only that some learners may need different types of learning activities for the objectives. Assessment also may indicate that some students have already attained certain clinical competencies and can progress to new areas of learning.

The second area of assessment relates to individual characteristics of students that may influence their learning and clinical performance. Students and nurses today represent a diverse group of learners with varied cultural backgrounds, learning styles, and other characteristics. The average age of nursing students has increased, and students bring with them a wealth of life and other experiences. In addition many students combine their nursing education with other role responsibilities, such as family and work. Information about these characteristics, among others, gives the teacher a better understanding of the students and their responses to different learning situations. Faculty members need to accept individual differences among students and use this knowledge in planning the learning activities.

Planning Clinical Learning Activities

Following assessment of learner needs and characteristics, the teacher plans and then delivers the instruction. In planning the learning activities, the main considerations are the competencies to be developed in the clinical practicum, or outcomes to be met in the clinical component of the course, and individual learner needs. Other factors, though, that influence decisions on clinical activities include the philosophy and outcomes of the nursing program, characteristics of the clinical setting, and teacher availability to guide learners.

Clinical Competencies/Outcomes of Clinical Practicum.   Clinical learning activities are selected to facilitate students' developing the essential competencies for clinical practice in that course or to meet the outcomes of the clinical practicum, depending on how these are stated by faculty members in the clinical course. The learning activities may include patient care assignment, but care of patients is not the only learning activity in which students engage in the practice setting. The specific competencies to be developed or outcomes to be achieved in that course should guide selection of learning activities. If the competencies focus on communication skills, then the learning activities may involve interviews with patients and families, papers analyzing those interactions, role play, and simulated patient–nurse interactions, rather than providing direct care.

Learner Needs.   While the clinical outcomes provide the framework for planning the learning activities, the other main consideration is the needs of the student. The activities should build on the student's present knowledge and skills and take into consideration other learner characteristics. Each student does not have to complete the same learning activities; the teacher is responsible for individualizing the clinical activities so that they best meet each student's needs while promoting achievement of the course outcomes.

Learning activities also build on one another. Planning includes organizing the activities to provide for the progressive development of knowledge and skills for each learner.

Philosophy and Outcomes of the Program.   The philosophy of the nursing program, in terms of the faculty's beliefs about learning, teaching, and clinical practice, ultimately influences the clinical activities planned for students. If the philosophy emphasizes self-direction and independence in learning, then opportunities should be provided in clinical practice for student choice of learning activities.

Clinical activities also should be consistent with the program outcomes. If one of the outcomes of the nursing program is development of critical thinking skill, then clinical activities need to promote critical thinking and decision making in clinical practice. Another program outcome may be use of research in clinical practice; this outcome suggests the need for learning activities in accessing, analyzing, and synthesizing research evidence and relating those findings to patient care.

Characteristics of the Clinical Setting.   The size of the agency, the patient population, the educational level and preparation of nurses and their availability and interest in working with students, other types of health care providers in the setting, and other characteristics of the clinical environment should be considered in planning the learning activities. These characteristics are taken into account when choosing an agency for use in a course, and they also guide the faculty in planning learning activities. In some settings certain activities may not be appropriate—patients may not be available or other resources may be lacking. In those instances a faculty member can plan clinical simulations for students to achieve the outcomes of the practicum.

Teacher Availability.   The teacher's availability to work with students in the clinical setting is an important consideration in planning the learning activities. Being available to students to guide their learning when needed is a characteristic of an effective clinical teacher. The number and level of students in a clinical group, for instance, may influence the type of learning activities planned for a course. Beginning students and nurses new to a clinical practice area may require more time and guidance from the teacher than experienced students and nurses. This principle is also important in distance education and other courses using preceptors; the preceptor or advanced practice nurse must be available to guide the students' learning in clinical practice.

Guiding Learners in Clinical Practice

The next step in the process of clinical teaching is that of guiding learners to acquire the essential knowledge, technological and other skills, and values for practice. Guiding reflects movement toward a destination where the way is unknown;

it is a facilitative and supportive process that leads the student toward achievement of the outcomes. Guiding is not supervision; supervision is a process of overseeing. Effective clinical teaching requires that the teacher guide students with their learning activities, not oversee their work.

This is the instructional phase in the clinical teaching process—the actual teaching of students in the clinical setting either on-site or at a distance. For distance education courses, the instructional phase may be carried out by preceptors, advanced practice nurses, and other providers depending on the course outcomes. With some learning activities, the teacher has a direct instructional role, for instance, demonstrating an intervention to students and questioning them to expand their understanding of a clinical situation. Other teaching activities, though, may be indirect, such as giving feedback on papers and preparing preceptors for their role, among others.

Murphy (2004) emphasized that clinical instruction is not only in the "content" being learned but also involves guiding students in learning "how to learn" and think about patient care. She found that focused reflection in clinical practice and articulation of thoughts in journals and postclinical conferences facilitated the development of students' clinical reasoning. With this process students become aware of their learning and thinking, recognizing their learning needs and developing skills needed for lifelong learning.

In the process of guiding learners, the teacher needs to be skilled in: (a) observing clinical performance, arriving at sound judgments about that performance, and planning additional learning activities if needed and (b) questioning students to promote critical thinking and higher level learning.

Skill in Observing Performance. Observing students as they carry out their clinical activities allows the teacher to identify continued areas of learning and when assistance is needed from the teacher. This information, in turn, suggests new learning activities for clinical practice.

Observations of students may be influenced by the teacher's values and biases, which may affect what they see as they observe a student's performance and their impressions of the quality of that performance. All educators should know their own values and biases that might influence their observations of student performance in clinical practice and judgments about student performance of the competencies.

Guidelines for observing students include the following

- examine own values and biases that may influence observations of students in clinical practice and judgments about clinical performance;

- do not rely on first impressions because these might change significantly with further observations of the student (Nitko, 2004);

- make a series of observations before drawing conclusions about clinical performance;

- share with students on a continual basis observations made of clinical performance and judgments about whether students are meeting the clinical competencies;

- focus observations on the outcomes of the clinical course or competencies to be achieved;

- when the observations reveal other aspects of performance that need further development, share these with students and use the information as a way of providing feedback on performance;

- discuss observations with students, obtain their perceptions of performance, and be willing to modify judgments when a different perspective is offered (Oermann & Gaberson, 2006).

Skill in Questioning Students. The second skill needed by the teacher to effectively guide clinical learning activities is ability to ask thought-provoking questions without students feeling that they are being interrogated. Open-ended questions about students' thinking and the rationale they used for arriving at clinical decisions foster development of critical thinking skills, an important outcome of clinical practice (Oermann, 1998; Oermann, Truesdell, & Ziolkowski, 2000; Profetto-McGrath, Smith, Day, & Yonge, 2004; Sedlak, & Doheny, 2004). Faculty, however, tend to ask questions that focus on recall of facts rather than ones that foster critical thinking (Profetto-McGrath et al., 2004). When questioning students in clinical practice, the teacher should assess understanding of relevant concepts and theories and how they apply to patient care. Other questions can ask students about different decisions possible in a clinical situation, consequences of each decision, the decision they would make, and their rationale; about different problems, possible interventions, and their evidence base; and about assumptions underlying their thinking (Oermann, 1998; Oermann et al., 2000). Questions should encourage learners to think beyond the obvious.

The way in which questions are asked is also significant. The purpose of questioning is to encourage students to consider other perspectives and possibilities, not to drill them and create added stress. In the beginning of a clinical course, and particularly in the beginning of the nursing program, the teacher should discuss the purpose of questioning and its relationship to developing critical thinking skills. The teacher can demonstrate the type of questions that will be asked in the course and how those questions encourage critical thinking.

Because questioning is for instructional purposes, students need to be comfortable that their responses will not influence their clinical grades. Instead, the questions asked and answers given are an essential part of the teaching process, to promote learning and development of critical thinking skills, not for grading purposes. Only with this framework will students be comfortable in responding to these higher-level questions and evaluating alternate perspectives, using the teacher as a resource. Collegial discussions promote reflection on practice competence and lead to developing clinical judgment (Weber, 2005).

Evaluating Clinical Learning and Performance

The remaining component of the clinical teaching process is evaluation. Clinical evaluation serves two purposes: formative and summative. Through formative evaluation the teacher monitors student progress toward meeting the outcomes of the clinical course and demonstrating competency in clinical practice. Formative evaluation provides information about further learning needs of students and where additional clinical instruction is needed. Clinical evaluation that is formative is not intended for grading purposes; instead, it is designed to diagnose learning needs as a basis for further instruction.

Summative evaluation, in contrast, takes place at the end of the learning process to ascertain if the course outcomes have been achieved and competencies developed (Oermann & Gaberson, 2006). Summative evaluation provides the basis for determining grades in clinical practice or certifying competency. It occurs at the completion of a course, an educational program, orientation, and other types of programs. This type of clinical evaluation determines what *has been* learned rather than what *can be* learned.

There are many clinical evaluation strategies that can be used in nursing courses. These are discussed and examples are provided in Chapter 16.

SUMMARY

Teaching is a complex process intended to facilitate learning. While the goal of teaching is to lead students in discovering knowledge for themselves, the teacher encourages this discovery through deliberate teaching actions that lead in that direction. The process of clinical teaching begins with identification of the goals and outcomes for clinical learning and proceeds through assessing the learner, planning clinical learning activities, guiding students, and evaluating clinical learning and performance. The goals and outcomes suggest areas for assessment, provide guidelines for teaching, and are the basis for evaluating learning. They may be expressed in the form of clinical objectives, outcomes, or competencies and may be established for an entire course or for specific clinical activities. The outcomes of clinical practice should be communicated clearly to students, in written form, and understood by them. Similarly, the teacher has an important responsibility in discussing these outcomes and related clinical activities with agency personnel.

Teaching begins at the level of the learner. The teacher's goal, therefore, is to assess the student's present level of knowledge and skill and other characteristics that may influence developing the clinical competencies. In the first area of assessment, data are collected on whether the student possesses the prerequisite knowledge and skills for the clinical situation at hand and for completing the learning activities. This assessment is important so that students engage in learning activities that build on their present knowledge and skills. When students lack the prerequisites, then the instruction can fill in and more efficiently move students forward in their learning. The second area of assessment relates to individual characteristics of students that may influence their learning and clinical performance, such as age, learning style, and cultural background.

Following assessment of learner needs and characteristics, the teacher plans and then delivers the instruction. In planning the learning activities, the main considerations are the objectives and individual learner needs. Other factors that influence decisions about clinical activities include the philosophy and outcomes of the nursing program, characteristics of the clinical setting, and teacher availability to guide learners.

The next step in the process of clinical teaching is that of guiding learners to acquire essential knowledge, skills, and values for practice. In this process of guiding learners, the teacher needs to be skilled in (a) observing clinical performance, arriving at sound judgments about that performance, and planning additional learning activities if needed and (b) questioning learners to encourage critical thinking, but without interrogating them.

The last component of the clinical teaching process is evaluation. Clinical evaluation can be formative or summative. Through formative evaluation the teacher monitors student progress in meeting the clinical outcomes and demonstrating competency in clinical practice. Clinical evaluation that is formative is not intended for grading purposes; instead, it is designed to diagnose learning needs as a basis for further instruction.

Summative evaluation, in contrast, takes place at the end of the learning period to ascertain if the outcomes have been achieved and competencies developed. It occurs at the completion of a course, an educational program, orientation, and other types of programs. This type of clinical evaluation determines what *has been* learned rather than what *can be* learned.

REFERENCES

Murphy, J. I. (2004). Using focused reflection and articulation to promote clinical reasoning: An evidence-based teaching strategy. *Nursing Education Perspectives, 25*, 226–231.

Murphy, J. I. (2005). How to learn, not what to learn: Three strategies that foster lifelong learning in clinical settings. In M. H. Oermann & K. T. Heinrich (Eds.), *Annual review of nursing education* (Vol. 3, pp. 37–55). New York: Springer Publishing.

Nitko, A. J. (2004). *Educational assessment of students* (4th ed.). Upper Saddle River, NJ: Pearson Prentice Hall.

Oermann, M. H. (1998). How to assess critical thinking in clinical practice. *Dimensions of Critical Care Nursing, 17*, 322–327.

Oermann, M. H. (2004). Using active learning in lecture: Best of "both worlds." *Journal of Nursing Education Scholarship, 1*(1), 1–11. Retrieved from http://www.bepress.com/ijnes/vol1/iss1/art1

Oermann, M. H., & Gaberson, K. B. (2006). *Evaluation and testing in nursing education* (2nd ed.). New York: Springer Publishing.

Oermann, M. H., Truesdell, S., & Ziolkowski, L. (2000). Strategy to assess, develop, and evaluate critical thinking. *Journal of Continuing Education in Nursing, 31*, 155–160.

Profetto-McGrath, J., Smith, K. B., Day, R. A., & Yonge, O. (2004). The questioning skills of tutors and students in a context based baccalaureate nursing program. *Nurse Education Today, 24*, 363–372.

Richardson, K., & Trudeau, K. J. (2003). A case for problem-based collaborative learning in the nursing classroom. *Nurse Educator, 26*, 83–88.

Sedlak, C. A., & Doheny, M. O. (2004). Critical thinking: What's new and how to foster thinking among nursing students. In M. H. Oermann & K. Heinrich (Eds.), *Annual review of nursing education* (Vol. 2, pp. 185–204). New York: Springer Publishing.

Weber, S. (2005). Promoting critical thinking in students. *Journal of the American Academy of Nurse Practitioners, 17*, 205–206.

Chapter 6

Ethical and Legal Issues in Clinical Teaching

Clinical teaching and learning take place in a social context. Teachers, students, staff members, and patients have roles, rights, and responsibilities that sometimes are in conflict. These conflicts create legal and ethical dilemmas for clinical teachers. This chapter discusses some ethical and legal issues related to clinical teaching and offers suggestions for preventing, minimizing, and managing these difficult situations.

ETHICAL ISSUES

Ethical standards make it possible for nurses, patients, teachers, and students to understand and respect each other. Contemporary bioethical standards include those related to respect for human dignity, autonomy, and freedom; beneficence; justice; veracity; privacy; and fidelity (Husted & Husted, 2001; Oermann & Gaberson, 2006; Williams, 2002). These standards are important considerations for all parties involved in clinical teaching and learning.

Learners in a Service Setting

If the word *clinical* means "involving direct observation of the patient," clinical activities must take place where patients are. Traditionally, learners encounter patients in health care service settings, such as acute care, extended care, and rehabilitation facilities. With the current focus on primary prevention, however, patients increasingly receive health care in home, community, and school environments (Stokes & Kost, 2004). Whatever the setting, patients are there to receive health care, staff members have the responsibility to provide care, and students are present to learn (Williams, 2002). Are these purposes always compatible?

Although it has been almost three decades since Corcoran (1977) raised ethical questions about the use of service settings for learning activities, those concerns are still valid. On the one hand, in the clinical setting, learners are nursing students or new staff members who are somewhat less skilled than experienced practitioners. Although their activities are observed and guided by clinical teachers, learners are not expected to provide cost-effective, efficient patient care services. On the other hand, patients expect quality service when they seek health care; providing learning opportunities for students usually is not a priority. The ethical standard of *beneficence* refers to the duty to help, to produce beneficial outcomes, or at least to do no harm (Husted & Husted, 2001). Is this standard violated when the learners' chief purpose for being in the clinical environment is to learn, not to give care?

Patients who encounter learners in clinical settings may feel exploited or fear invasion of their privacy; they may receive care that takes more time and creates more discomfort than if provided by expert practitioners. The presence of learners in a clinical setting also requires more time and energy of staff members, who usually are expected to give and receive reports from students, answer their questions, and demonstrate or help with patient care. These activities may divert staff members' attention from their primary responsibility for patient care, interfere with their efficient performance, and affect their satisfaction with their work (Corcoran, 1977).

Because achieving the desired outcomes of clinical teaching requires learning activities in real service settings, teachers must consider the rights and needs of learners, patients, and staff members when planning clinical learning activities. The clinical teacher is responsible for making the learning objectives clear to all involved persons and for ensuring that learning activities do not prevent achievement of service goals. Patients should receive adequate information about the presence of learners before giving their informed consent to participate in clinical learning activities. The teacher should assure the learners' preparation and readiness for clinical learning as well as his or her own presence and competence as an instructor, as discussed in Chapter 3.

Student–Faculty Relationships

Respect for Persons.   As discussed in Chapter 1, an effective and beneficial relationship between clinical teacher and student is built on a base of mutual trust and respect. Although both parties are responsible for maintaining this relationship, the clinical teacher must initiate it by demonstrating trust and respect for students. A trusting, respectful relationship with students demonstrates the teacher's commitment to ethical values of respect for human dignity and autonomy.

In a classic study of nursing students' perceptions of unethical teaching behaviors (Theis, 1988), 50% of the incidents described by students occurred in clinical settings, as compared with 39% in the classroom. Of the clinical incidents, 58% were classified as violations of respect for persons. Examples of such behavior included questioning and criticizing students in public areas, talking about a patient in the patient's presence, and allowing students to observe a catheterization without asking the patient's permission. As these examples illustrate, a clinical teacher's failure to model respect for patients can also be considered an unethical teaching behavior. Theis pointed out that in some instances, the teacher's behavior may have been misinterpreted by students. For example, while the student believed that the instructor failed to seek the patient's consent to the presence of observers, the instructor may have done so when the student was not present. However, if the teacher had obtained consent, pointing this out to the student would have been prevented the misunderstanding as well as reinforced the ethical value of respect for persons (Theis, 1988).

A recently published case study (Lewenson, Truglio-Londrigan, & Singleton, 2005) identified similar issues related to an incident of ethical violation in a classroom setting. While the initial focus was on the student's breach of conduct, the faculty members recognized issues related to their own ethical conduct and how they modeled that behavior to students. The importance of teaching and practicing ethical conduct in academic settings was emphasized.

Fairness and Justice. The ethical standard of *justice* refers to fair treatment — judging each person's behavior by the same standards. Clinical teachers must evaluate each student's performance by the same standard. Students may perceive a clinical teacher's behavior as unfair when the teacher appears to favor some students by praising, supporting, and offering better learning opportunities to them more than others (Theis, 1988). Teachers who develop social relationships with some students are more likely to be perceived as unfair by other students. The teacher's relationships with students should be collegial and collaborative without being overly personal and social (Johnson & Halstead, 2005).

Students' Privacy Rights

When students have a succession of clinical instructors, it is common for the instructors to communicate information about student performance. Learning about the students' levels of performance in their previous clinical assignment helps the next instructor to anticipate their needs and to plan appropriate learning activities for them. Although students usually benefit when teachers share such information about their learning needs, personal information that students reveal in confidence should *not* be shared with other teachers. Additionally, when sharing information about students, teachers should focus on factual statements about performance without adding their personal judgments. Characterizing or labeling students is rarely helpful to the next instructor, and such behavior violates ethical standards of privacy as well as respect for persons.

Because clinical teachers in nursing education programs are themselves professional nurses, they sometimes experience conflict regarding their knowledge of students' health problems. As nurses, they would tend to respond in a therapeutic way if a student revealed personal information about a health concern, but as teachers, their primary obligation is to a teacher–student relationship. Absent any existing institutional policy or compelling evidence that the personal information should be disclosed to protect the safety of the student or other person, educators should follow the principle of what action would best promote student learning (Morgan, 2001).

Competent Teaching

Applying the ethical standard of beneficence to teaching, students have a right to expect that their clinical teachers are competent, responsible, and knowledgeable. As discussed in Chapter 4, clinical competence, including expert knowledge and clinical skill, is an essential characteristic of effective clinical teachers. In addition, clinical teachers must be competent in (1) facilitating and supporting students in their learning activities, including planning assignments that assist students to apply knowledge to practice, promoting student independence, and asking and answering questions; (2) evaluating student performance, including giving specific, timely feedback; and (3) communicating effectively with students, including developing collegial relationships with them (Stokes & Kost, 2004). Examples of unethical behavior related to clinical teacher competence include not being available for guidance in the clinical setting and demonstrating or directing a student to perform a skill in a manner that violated aseptic technique (Theis, 1988).

Academic Dishonesty

Although cheating and other forms of dishonest behavior are believed to be common in the classroom environment, academic dishonesty can occur in clinical settings as well. *Academic dishonesty* is defined as intentional participation in deceptive practices regarding the academic work of self or others. Dishonest acts include lying, cheating, plagiarizing, altering or forging records, falsely representing oneself, and knowingly assisting another person to commit a dishonest act (Bradshaw & Lowenstein, 1999; Gaberson, 1997).

Cheating is the use of unauthorized help in completing an academic assignment. An example of cheating is copying portions of a classmate's case study analysis and presenting the assignment as one's own work. Similarly, the student who asks a staff member's assistance to calculate a medication dose but tells the instructor that he or she did the work alone also is cheating (Bradshaw & Lowenstein, 1999; Gaberson, 1997).

Other examples of academic dishonesty in the clinical setting include the following:

- *Lying.* A student tells the instructor that she attempted a home visit to a patient but the patient was not at home. In fact, the student overslept and missed the scheduled time of the visit.

- *Plagiarism.* While preparing materials for a patient teaching project, a student paraphrases portions of a published teaching pamphlet without citing the source.

- *Altering a document.* A staff nurse orientee adds additional information to the documentation of nursing care for a patient on the previous day.

- *False representation.* As a family nurse practitioner student begins a physical examination, the patient addresses the student as "Doctor." The student continues with the examination and does not tell the patient that he is a nurse.

- *Assisting another in a dishonest act.* Student A asks Student B to cover for her while she leaves the clinical agency to run a personal errand. The teacher asks Student B if he has seen Student A; Student B says that he thinks she has accompanied a patient to the physical therapy department.

While some of the previous examples may appear to be harmless or minor infractions, dishonest acts should be taken seriously because they can have harmful effects on patients, learners, faculty–student relationships, and the educational program. Clinical dishonesty can jeopardize patient safety if learners fail to report errors or do not receive adequate guidance because their competence is assumed. Mutual trust forms the basis for effective teacher–learner relationships, and academic dishonesty can damage a teacher's trust in students. Dishonesty that is ignored by teachers conveys the impression to students that this behavior is acceptable, and honest students resent teachers who fail to deal effectively with cheating. An educational program's reputation can be damaged when agency staff members discover clinical errors that have been concealed by students and not addressed by teachers; the result may be the loss of that agency for future clinical activities (Gaberson, 1997).

Clinical academic dishonesty usually results from one or more of the following factors:

- *Competition, desire for good grades, and heavy workload.* Competition for good grades in clinical nursing courses may result from student misunderstanding of the evaluation framework. If students believe that a limited number of good grades is available, they may compete fiercely with their classmates. Competition may lead to deceptive acts in an attempt to earn higher grades than other students. Additionally, many nursing students have other pressures related to employment and family responsibilities; they may feel overloaded and unable to meet all of the demands of a rigorous nursing education program without resorting to cheating (Bradshaw & Lowenstein, 1999).
- *Emphasis on perfection.* As discussed in Chapter 2, clinical teachers often communicate the expectation that good nurses do not make mistakes. Although nursing education attempts to prepare practitioners who will perform carefully and skillfully, a standard of perfection is unrealistic (Gaberson, 1997). Students naturally make mistakes in the process of learning new knowledge and skills, and punishment for mistakes, in the form of low grades or a negative performance evaluation, will not prevent these errors. In fact, it is the fear of punishment that often motivates students to conceal errors, and errors that are not reported are often harmful to patient safety (Kohn, Corrigan, & Donaldson 2000).
- *Poor role modeling.* The influence of role models on behavior is strong. Nursing students and novice staff nurses who observe dishonest behavior of teachers and experienced staff members may emulate these examples, especially when the dishonest acts have gone unnoticed, unreported, or unpunished.

Clinical teachers can use a variety of approaches to discourage academic dishonesty. They should be exemplary role models of honest behavior for learners to emulate (Bradshaw & Lowenstein, 1999). They should acknowledge that mistakes occur in the learning process and create a learning climate that allows students to make mistakes in a safe environment with guidance and feedback for problem solving. However, students need reassurance that, if humanly possible, teachers will not allow them to make errors that would harm patients. Finally, each nursing education program should develop a policy that defines academic dishonesty and specifies appropriate penalties for violations. This policy should be communicated to all students, reviewed with them at regular intervals, and applied consistently and fairly to every violation (Gaberson, 1997).

When enforcing the academic integrity policy, it is important to apply ethical standards to protect the dignity and privacy of students. A public accusation of dishonesty that is found later to be ungrounded can damage a student's reputation. The teacher should speak with the student privately and calmly, describe the student's behavior and the teacher's interpretation of it, and provide the student with an opportunity to respond to the charge. It is essential to keep an open mind until all available evidence is evaluated because the student may be able to supply a reasonable explanation for the behavior that the teacher interpreted as cheating (Gaberson, 1997).

LEGAL ISSUES

It is beyond the scope of this book to discuss and interpret all federal, state, and local laws that have implications for clinical teaching and evaluation, and the authors are not qualified to give legal advice to clinical teachers regarding their practice. It is recommended that clinical teachers refer questions about the legal implications of policies and procedures to the legal counsel for the institution in which they are employed; concerns about a teacher's legal rights in a specific situation are best referred to the individual's attorney. However, this section of the chapter discusses common legal issues that often arise in the practice of clinical teaching

Students With Disabilities

Two federal laws have implications for the education of learners with disabilities. The Rehabilitation Act of 1973, Section 504, prohibits public postsecondary institutions that receive federal funding from denying access or participation to individuals with disabilities. The Americans with Disabilities Act (ADA) of 1990 guarantees persons with disabilities equal access to educational opportunities if they are otherwise qualified for admission (Frank & Halstead, 2005). An individual who has a physical or mental impairment that substantially limits one or more of that individual's major life activities, and that the individual has a record of, is regarded as having such impairment (Brent, 2004b). In nursing education programs, qualified individuals with disabilities are those who meet the essential eligibility requirements for participation, with or without modifications (Southern Regional Education Board [SREB], 2004).

A common goal of nursing education programs is to produce graduates who can function safely and competently in the roles for which they were prepared. For this reason, it is appropriate for those who make admission decisions to determine whether applicants could reasonably be expected to develop the necessary competence. The first step in this decision process is to define the core performance standards necessary for participation in the program. Because nursing is a practice discipline, core performance standards include cognitive, sensory, affective, and psychomotor competencies. The SREB recommended that such lists of core performance standards be shared with all applicants to nursing education programs to allow them to make initial judgments about their qualifications (SREB, 2004).

Persons with disabilities who are admitted to nursing education programs are responsible for informing the institution of the disability and requesting reasonable accommodations (Brent, 2004b). Each nursing education program must determine on an individual basis whether the necessary modifications can reasonably be made. Reasonable accommodations for participating in clinical learning activities might include

- allowing additional time for a student with a qualified learning disability to complete an assignment;

- allowing additional time to complete the program;

- scheduling clinical learning activities in facilities that are readily accessible to and usable by individuals who use wheelchairs or crutches;

- providing the use of an amplified stethoscope for a student with a hearing impairment.

Reasonable accommodations do not include lowering academic standards or eliminating essential technical performance requirements. However, nurse educators need to distinguish essential from traditional functions by discussing such philosophical issues as to whether individuals who will never practice bedside nursing in the conventional manner should be admitted to nursing education programs (Frank & Halstead, 2005).

Due Process

Another legal issue related to clinical teaching is that of student rights to due process. In educational settings, due process requires that students be informed of the standards by which their performance will be judged, that they will receive timely feedback about their performance, and that they will have an opportunity to correct behavior that does not meet standards. In other words, learners have the right to be informed of their academic deficiencies, how those deficiencies will affect their academic progress, and what they need to do to correct the problem (Brent, 2004a; Johnson & Halstead, 2005). Students who experience academic failure or dismissal from a nursing education program often appeal these decisions on the basis of denial of due process.

The 14th Amendment of the United States Constitution specifies that the state cannot deprive a person of life, liberty, or property without due process of law. With regard to the rights of students to due process, however, this constitutional protection extends only to those enrolled in public institutions. Students at private institutions instead may base a claim against the school on discrimination or contract law. For example, if a private school publishes a code of student rights and procedures for student grievances in its student handbook, those documents may be regarded as part of a contract between the school and the student. In paying and accepting tuition, the student and the school jointly agree to abide by this code of rights and set of procedures. A student may sue on the basis of breach of contract if the school does not follow the stated due process procedures (Brent, 2004a; Johnson & Halstead, 2005).

Courts hold different standards for due process based on whether it applies to academic or disciplinary decisions. Academic decisions include assigning a failing grade in a course, delaying progress, and dismissal from a program because of failure to maintain acceptable academic standing. The courts traditionally have been reluctant to intervene in academic decisions, believing that the faculty is competent to judge student performance according to academic criteria or objectives (Brent, 2004a). Thus, academic due process is viewed by the courts as substantive due process, and the following procedures are generally sufficient:

- Students are informed in advance about the academic standards that will be used to judge their performance and about the process for appealing such decisions.

- Students are notified about the potential for academic failure well before grading decisions are made. Ideally, notification occurs orally and in writing, and the teacher and student work together to determine a plan for overcoming the deficiencies.

- Student performance is evaluated using the stated standards or criteria, and grades are assigned according to the stated policy.

- If a student believes that a grade or other academic decision is unfair, the stated appeal or grievance process is followed. Usually, the first level of appeal is to the teacher or group of faculty who assigned the grade. If the conflict is not resolved at that level, the student usually has the right of appeal to the administrator to whom the teacher reports. The next level of appeal is usually to a student standing committee or appeal panel of nursing faculty members. Finally, the student should have the right to appeal the decision to the highest level administrator in the nursing program.

Of course, if students exhaust every level of appeal and are still not satisfied with the outcome, they have the right to seek relief in the court system. It is important to note that the courts will allow such a lawsuit to go forward only if there is evidence that the student has first exhausted all internal school remedies. However, if the educational program faculty and administrators have followed substantive due process procedures as previously described, it is unlikely that the academic decision will be reversed. If the student appeals to a court of law, the burden of proof that academic due process was denied rests with the student. With regard to due process for academic decisions, the key to resolving conflict and minimizing faculty liability is in maintaining communication with students whose performance is not meeting standards (Brent, 2004a; Johnson & Halstead, 2004).

Disciplinary decisions such as dismissal on the basis of misconduct or dishonesty require a higher level of due process, called procedural due process. *Procedural due process* guarantees the right to a hearing before dismissal. Components of disciplinary due process include the following:

• The student is provided with adequate written notice including specific details concerning the misconduct. For example, a notice may inform the student that she failed to attend a required clinical activity; that neither the faculty member or nursing unit secretary was informed of the anticipated absence, in violation of school policy on professional conduct; and that because this incident represented the third violation of professional conduct standards, the student would be dismissed from the program, according to the sanctions provided in the policy.

• The student is provided the opportunity for a fair, impartial hearing on the charges. The student has the right to speak on his or her own behalf, to present witnesses and evidence, and to question the other participants in the case (usually teachers and administrators). Using the preceding example, the student might present evidence that she did attempt to call the faculty member to report her absence; this evidence could include the date and time of the call, the name of the person with whom she spoke, and a copy of a telephone bill with the toll call charge. Although the student and the faculty member are entitled to the advice of legal counsel, neither attorney may question or cross-examine witnesses.

If the decision of the hearing panel is to uphold the dismissal, the student has the right to seek remedy from the court system if he or she believes that due process was not followed. However, in disciplinary cases, the burden of proof that due process was denied rests with the student.

Negligence, Liability, and Unsafe Clinical Practice

When determining whether a given action meets the criteria for professional negligence, the overall standard of care is what an ordinary, reasonable, and prudent person would have done in the same context. The standard of care for a nursing student is not what another nursing student would have done; students are held to the same standards of care as registered nurses (Brent, 2004b). The concept of personal liability also applies to cases of professional negligence. Each person is responsible for his or her own behavior, including negligent acts. Students are liable for their own actions as long as they are performing according to the usual standard of care for their education and experience, and they seek guidance when they are uncertain what to do. Therefore, it is not true that students practice under the faculty member's license (Brent, 2004b).

Teachers are not liable for negligent acts performed by their students as long as the teacher has (1) selected appropriate learning activities based on objectives, (2) determined that students have prerequisite knowledge, skills, and attitudes necessary to complete their assignments, and (3) provided competent guidance. However, teachers are liable for their negligent actions if they make assignments that require more knowledge and skill than the learner has developed, or if they fail to guide student activities appropriately.

If a student demonstrates clinical performance that potentially is unsafe, the student and the teacher who made the assignment may be liable for any subsequent injury to the patient. However, because time for learning must precede time for evaluation, is it fair for the teacher to remove the student from the clinical area when to do so would prevent the student's access to learning opportunities for which he or she has paid tuition? In this case, denying access to clinical learning activities because of unsafe practice should not be considered an academic grading decision. Instead, it is an appropriate response to protecting the rights of patients to safe, competent care.

The teacher's failure to take such protective action potentially places the teacher and the educational program at risk for liability. Instead of denying the student access to all learning opportunities, removal from the clinical setting should be followed by a substitute assignment that would help the student to remove the deficiency in knowledge, skill, or attitude. For example, the student might be given a library assignment to acquire the information necessary to guide safe patient care, or an extra skills laboratory session could be arranged to allow more practice of psychomotor skills. A set of standards on safe clinical practice and a school policy that enforces the standards are helpful guides to faculty decision making and action while protecting student and faculty rights. Table 6.1 is an example of safe clinical practice standards, and Table 6.2 is an example of a policy that enforces these standards.

TABLE 6.1   Standards of Safe Clinical Practice

XXXXXX UNIVERSITY
SCHOOL OF NURSING
BSN PROGRAM

Standards of Safe Clinical Practice

In clinical practice, students are expected to demonstrate responsibility and accountability as professional nurses with the goal of health promotion and prevention of harm to self and others. The School of Nursing believes that this goal will be attained if each student's clinical practice adheres to the Standards of Safe Clinical Practice. Safe clinical performance always includes, but is not limited to, the following behaviors:

1. Practice within boundaries of the nursing student role and the scope of practice of the registered professional nurse.
2. Comply with institutional policies and procedures for implementing nursing care.
3. Prepare for clinical learning assignments according to course requirements and as determined for the specific clinical setting.
4. Demonstrate the application of previously learned skills and principles in providing nursing care.
5. Promptly report significant client information in a clear, accurate, and complete oral or written manner to the appropriate person or persons.

Acknowledgment

I have read the XXXXXX University School of Nursing Standards of Safe Clinical Practice and I agree to adhere to them. I understand that these standards are expectations for my clinical practice and will be incorporated into the evaluation of my clinical performance in all clinical courses. Failure to meet these standards may result in my removal from the clinical area, which may result in clinical failure.

_____

Signature and Date

TABLE 6.2   Policy on Safe Clinical Practice

XXXXXX UNIVERSITY
SCHOOL OF NURSING
BSN PROGRAM

Safe Clinical Practice Policy

POLICY:
During enrollment in the XXXXXX University School of Nursing BSN Program, all students, in all clinical activities, are expected to adhere to the Standards of Safe Clinical Practice. Failure to abide by these standards will result in disciplinary action, which may include dismissal from the nursing program.

PROCEDURES:
1. Students will receive a copy of the Standards of Safe Clinical Practice, and they will be reviewed during the Annual Nursing Assembly at the beginning of each academic year. At that time, students will be required to sign an Agreement to adhere to the standards. Each student will retain one copy of the Agreement and one copy will be filed in the student's file.
2. Violation of these Standards will result in the following disciplinary action:
   a. First Violation
      (1) Student will be given an immediate oral warning by the faculty member. The incident will be documented by the faculty member on the *Violation of Standards of Safe Clinical Practice* form. One copy of this form will be given to the student and one copy will be kept in the student's record.
      (2) At the discretion of the faculty member, the student may be required to leave the clinical unit for the remainder of that day. The student may be given an alternative assignment.
      (3) If this violation is of a serious nature, it may be referred to the Associate Dean and the Dean of Nursing for further disciplinary action as in b. and c. below.
   b. Second Violation
      (1) The faculty member will document the incident on the *Violation of Safe Clinical Practice* form. Following discussion of the incident with the student, the faculty member will forward a copy of the form to the Associate Dean for review and recommendation regarding further action.
      (2) The recommendation of the Associate Dean will be forwarded to the Dean of Nursing for review and decision regarding reprimand or dismissal. This disciplinary action process will be documented and placed in the student's record.
   c. If the student has not been dismissed and remains in the Program following the above disciplinary action, any additional violation will be documented and referred as above to the Associate Dean and the Dean of Nursing for disciplinary action, which may include dismissal from the Program.
   d. The rights of students will be safeguarded as set forth in the XXXXXX University *Code of Student Rights, Responsibilities, and Conduct* published in the current *XXXXXX University Student Handbook.*

Documentation and Record Keeping

Teachers should keep records of their evaluations of student clinical performance. These records may include anecdotal notes, summaries of faculty–student conferences, progress reports, and summative clinical evaluations. These records are helpful in documenting that students received feedback about their performance, areas of teacher concern, and information about student progress toward correcting deficiencies (Case & Oermann, 2004).

An *anecdotal note* is a narrative description of the observed behavior of the student, in relation to a specific learning objective. The note also may include the teacher's interpretation of the behavior, recorded separately from the description. Limiting the description and optional interpretation to a specified clinical objective avoids recording extraneous information, which is an ineffective use of the teacher's time. Anecdotal notes should record both positive and negative behaviors so as not to give the impression that the teacher is biased against the student. Students should review these notes and have an opportunity to comment on them; used in this way, anecdotal notes are an effective means of communicating formative evaluation information to students (Case & Oermann, 2004). Some sources recommend that both teacher and student sign the notes.

Writing anecdotal notes for every student, every day, is unnecessarily time-consuming. An effective, efficient approach might be to specify a minimum number of notes to be written for each student in relation to specified objectives. A student whose performance is either meritorious or cause for concern might prompt the instructor to write more numerous notes.

Records of student–teacher conferences, or *conference notes*, likewise are summaries of discussions that focused on areas of concern, plans to address deficiencies, and progress toward correcting weaknesses. These conferences should take place in privacy and should address the teacher's responsibility to protect patient safety, concern about the student's clinical deficiencies, and a sincere desire to assist the student to improve. During the conference, the student also has opportunities to clarify and respond to the teacher's feedback. At times, an objective third party such as a department chairperson or program director may be asked to participate in the conference to witness and clarify the comments of both teacher and student. The conference note should record the date, time, and place of the conference; the names and roles of participants; and a summary of the discussion, recommendations, and plans. The note may be signed only by the teacher or by all participants, according to institutional policy or guidelines (Johnson & Halstead, 2005).

Because they contain essentially formative evaluation information, anecdotal notes and conference notes should not be kept in the student's permanent record. Teachers should keep these records in their private files, taking appropriate precautions to ensure their security, until there is no reasonable expectation that they will be needed. In most cases, when the learner successfully completes the program or withdraws in good academic standing, these records can be discarded (again, taking appropriate security precautions). It is unlikely that successful learners will appeal favorable academic decisions. However, it is recommended that anecdotal records and conference notes be kept for longer periods when there is a chance that the learner may appeal the grade or other decision. The statute of limitations for such an appeal is a useful guide to a deciding how long to keep those materials. It is recommended that teachers consult with legal counsel if there is a question as to institutional policy on retention of records.

SUMMARY

Because clinical teaching and learning take place in a social context, the rights of teachers, students, staff members, and patients are sometimes in conflict. These conflicts create legal and ethical dilemmas for clinical teachers. This chapter discussed some ethical and legal issues related to clinical teaching.

Ethical standards such as respect for human dignity, autonomy, and freedom; beneficence; justice; veracity; privacy; and fidelity are important considerations for all parties involved in clinical teaching and learning. Students must learn to apply these standards to nursing practice, and teachers must apply them in their relationships with students as well as their teaching and evaluation responsibilities.

Specific ethical issues related to clinical teaching and learning include the presence of learners in a service setting, the need for faculty–student relationships to be based on justice and respect for persons, students' privacy rights, teaching competence, and academic dishonesty. Legal issues that have implications for clinical teaching and learning include educating students with disabilities, student rights to due process for academic and disciplinary decisions, standards of safe clinical practice, student and teacher negligence and liability, and documentation and record keeping regarding students' clinical performance.

Suggestions were offered for preventing, minimizing, and managing these difficult ethical and legal situations. Laws and institutional policies often provide guidelines for action in specific cases. However, these suggestions should not be construed as legal advice, and teachers are advised to seek legal counsel in regard to specific questions or problems.

REFERENCES

Bradshaw, M. J., & Lowenstein, A. (1999). Academic dishonesty: Addressing the problems of cheating, plagiarism, and professional misconduct. In K. R. Stevens & V. R. Cassidy (Eds.), *Evidence-based teaching: Current research in nursing education* (pp. 105–134). New York: National League for Nursing.

Brent, N. J. (2004a). The law and the nurse educator: A look at legal cases. In L. Caputi & L. Engelmann (Eds.), *Teaching nursing: The art and science* (pp. 813–846). Glen Ellyn, IL: College of DuPage Press.

Brent, N. J. (2004b). The law and the nursing student: Answers you will want to know. In L. Caputi & L. Engelmann (Eds.), *Teaching nursing: The art and science* (pp. 847–860). Glen Ellyn, IL: College of DuPage Press.

Case, B., & Oermann, M. H. (2004). Teaching in a clinical setting. In L. Caputi & L. Engelmann (Eds.), *Teaching nursing: The art and science* (pp. 126–177). Glen Ellyn, IL: College of DuPage Press.

Corcoran, S. (1977). Should a service setting be used as a learning laboratory? An ethical question. *Nursing Outlook, 25,* 771–774.

Frank, B., & Halstead, J. A. (2005). Teaching students with disabilities. In D. M. Billings & J. A. Halstead (Eds.), *Teaching in nursing: A guide for faculty* (2nd ed., pp. 67–86). St. Louis: Elsevier Saunders.

Gaberson, K. B. (1997). Academic dishonesty. *Nursing Forum, 32,* 14–20.

Husted, G. L., & Husted, J. H. (2001). *Ethical decision making in nursing: The symphonological approach* (3rd ed.). New York: Springer Publishing.

Johnson, E. G., & Halstead, J. A. (2005). The academic performance of students: Legal and ethical issues. In D. M. Billings & J. A. Halstead (Eds.), *Teaching in nursing: A guide for faculty* (2nd ed., pp. 41–66). St. Louis: Elsevier Saunders.

Kohn, L., Corrigan, J., & Donaldson, M. (2000). *To err is human: Building a safer health system.* Washington, DC: National Academy Press, Institute of Medicine.

Lewenson, S. B., Truglio-Londrigan, M., & Singleton, J. (2005). Practice what you teach: A case study of ethical conduct in the academic setting. *Journal of Professional Nursing, 21,* 89–96.

Morgan, J. E. (2001). Confidential student information in nursing education. *Nurse Educator, 26,* 289–292.

Oermann, M. H., & Gaberson, K. B. (2006). *Evaluation and testing in nursing education* (2nd ed.). New York: Springer Publishing.

Southern Regional Education Board. (2004). *The Americans with Disabilities Act: Implications for nursing education.* Retrieved June 28, 2006, from http://www.sreb.org/programs/nursing/publications/adareport.asp

Stokes, L., & Kost, G. (2005). Teaching in the clinical setting. In D. M. Billings & J. A. Halstead, (Eds.), *Teaching in nursing: A guide for faculty* (2nd ed., pp. 325–348). St. Louis: Elsevier Saunders.

Theis, E. C. (1988). Nursing students' perspectives of unethical teaching behaviors. *Journal of Nursing Education, 27,* 102–106.

Williams, M. D. (2002). Fidelity and obligation in faculty practice. *Journal of Professional Nursing, 18,* 247–248.

Chapter 7

Choosing Clinical Learning Assignments

One of the most important responsibilities of a clinical teacher is selecting clinical assignments related to outcomes that are appropriate to students' levels of knowledge and skill and yet challenging enough to motivate learning. Although directing a learner to provide comprehensive nursing care to one or more patients is a typical clinical assignment, it is only one of many possible assignments, and not always the most appropriate choice. This chapter presents a framework for selecting clinical learning assignments and discusses several alternatives to the traditional total patient care assignment.

PATIENT CARE VERSUS LEARNING ACTIVITY

When planning assignments, clinical teachers typically speak of "selecting patients" for whom students will care. However, as discussed in Chapter 1, the primary role of the nursing student in the clinical area is that of learner, not nurse. While it is true that nursing students need contact with patients to apply classroom learning to clinical practice, caring for patients is not synonymous with learning. Nursing students are *learning to care* for patients; they are not nurses with *responsibility for patient care* (Infante, 1985). Providing patient care does not guarantee transfer of knowledge from the classroom to clinical practice; instead, it often reflects work requirements of the clinical agency (Karuhije, 1997).

Many faculty members assume that caring for patients always constitutes a clinical assignment for students on every level of the nursing education program. Even in their earliest clinical courses, nursing students typically have responsibility for patient care while learning basic psychomotor and communication skills.

However, beginning-level nursing students are not ready to care for the typical patient in contemporary acute care settings, and this early responsibility for patient care often creates anxiety that interferes with learning.

As discussed in Chapter 2, changes in health care, technology, society, and education influence the competencies needed for professional nursing practice. Learning outcomes necessary for safe competent nursing practice today include cognitive skills of problem solving, decision making, and critical thinking, in addition to technical proficiency. If nurse educators are to produce creative, independent, assertive, and decisive practitioners, they cannot assume that students will acquire these competencies through patient care assignments. To produce these outcomes, clinical teachers should choose clinical assignments from a variety of learning activities, including participation in patient care.

FACTORS AFFECTING SELECTION
OF CLINICAL ASSIGNMENTS

The selection of learning activities within the context of the clinical teaching process is discussed in Chapter 5. Clinical activities help learners to apply knowledge to practice, develop skills, and cultivate professional values. Clinical assignments should be selected according to criteria such as the learning objectives of the clinical activity, needs of patients, availability and variety of learning opportunities in the clinical environment, and the needs, interests, and abilities of learners (Case & Oermann, 2004; Stokes & Kost, 2004).

Learning Outcomes

The most important criterion for the selection of clinical assignments is usually the desired learning outcome. The teacher should structure each clinical activity carefully in terms of the learning objectives, and each clinical activity should be an integral part of the course or educational program.

It is essential that the instructor, students, and staff members understand the goals of each clinical activity. Depending on the level of the learner, students may have difficulty envisioning how broad program or course outcomes can be achieved in the context of a specific clinical environment. It is the instructor's role to translate these outcomes into specific clinical objectives and to select and structure learning activities so that they relate logically and sequentially to the goals (Case & Oermann, 2004).

Learner Characteristics

As discussed in Chapter 5, the learner's educational level or previous experience, aptitude for learning, learning style, and specific needs, interests, and abilities also should influence the selection of clinical assignments. The teacher must consider these individual differences; all learners do not have the same needs, so it is unreasonable to expect them to have the same learning assignments on any given day (Case & Oermann, 2004).

For example, Student A learns skills at a slower pace than other students at the same level. The instructor should plan assignments so that this student has many opportunities for repetition of skills with feedback. If the objective is to learn the skills of medication administration, most students might be able to learn those skills in a reasonable amount of time in the context of providing care to one or more patients. Student A might learn more effectively with an assignment to administer all medications to a larger group of patients over the period of 1 day or more, without other patient care responsibilities. When the student has acquired the necessary level of skill, the next clinical assignment might be to administer medications while learning other aspects of care for one or more patients.

Students who are able to achieve the objectives of the essential curriculum (see Chapter 1) rather quickly might receive assignments from the enrichment curriculum that allow them to focus on their individual needs. For example, a student who is interested in perioperative nursing might be assigned to follow a patient through a surgical procedure, providing preoperative care, observing or participating in the surgery, assisting in immediate postoperative care in the postanesthesia care unit, and presenting a plan of care for home care in a postclinical conference.

Needs of Patients

Patient needs and care requirements should also be considered when planning clinical assignments for students. In relation to the learning objective, will the nursing care activities present enough of a challenge to the learner? Are they too complex for the learner to manage?

Even if patients signed consents for admission to the health care facility that included an agreement to the participation of learners in their care, their wishes regarding student assignment and those of their family members should be respected (Case & Oermann, 2004). At times of crisis, patients and family members may not wish to initiate a new nurse–patient relationship with a nursing student or new employee orientee. Nursing staff members who have provided care to these patients can often help the clinical teacher determine if student learning needs and specific patient and family needs both can be met through a particular clinical assignment.

Timing of Activities and Availability of Learning Opportunities

Because the purpose of clinical learning is to foster application of theory to practice, clinical learning activities should be related to what is being taught in the classroom. Ideally, clinical activities are scheduled concurrently with relevant classroom content so that learners can make immediate transfer and application of knowledge to nursing practice. However, there is little evidence of a relationship between clinical learning outcomes and the structure, timing, and organization of clinical learning activities (Dunn, Stockhausen, Thornton, & Barnard, 1995; Stokes & Kost, 2004).

The availability of learning opportunities to allow students to meet objectives often affects clinical assignments. The usual schedule of activities in the clinical facility may determine the optimum timing of learning activities. For example, if the learning objective for a new nursing student is "Identifies sources of information about patient needs from the health record," it would be difficult for students to gain access to patient records at the beginning or end of a shift. Thus, scheduling learners to arrive at the clinical site at mid-morning may allow better access to the resources necessary for learning.

Some clinical settings, such as outpatient clinics and operating rooms, are available both to patients and students only on a daytime, Monday through Friday schedule. In other settings, however, scheduling clinical learning assignments during evening or night hours or on weekend days may offer students better opportunities to meet certain objectives. If the learning objective is, "Implements health teaching for the parents of a premature or ill neonate," the best time for students to encounter parents may be during evening visiting hours or on weekends. Using these time periods for clinical activities may also avoid two or more groups of learners from different educational programs being in the same clinical area simultaneously, affecting the availability of learning opportunities.

Of course, planning learning activities at such times may potentially conflict with family, work, and other academic schedules and commitments for both teachers and students (Dunn et al., 1995; Stokes & Kost, 2004). In some cases (for example, with the use of preceptors) it is not necessary for the teacher to be present in the clinical setting with learners, thereby allowing more flexible scheduling of clinical activities.

OPTIONS FOR LEARNING ASSIGNMENTS

The creative teacher may select clinical assignments from a wide variety of learning activities. Several options for making assignments are discussed here.

Teacher-Selected or Learner-Selected Assignments

Although it is the teacher's responsibility to specify the learning objective, learners should have choices of learning activities that will help them achieve the objective. With learning outcomes such as assertiveness, creativity, independence, problem solving, and critical thinking, teachers must allow learners to participate actively in selecting their own clinical activities. Allowing learners to participate in selecting their own assignments may also reduce student anxiety.

Of course, the teacher should offer guidance in selecting appropriate learning activities through questions or comments that require students to evaluate their own needs, interests, and abilities. Sometimes teachers need to be more directive; a student may choose an assignment that clearly requires more knowledge or skill than the student has developed. In this case, the teacher must intervene to protect patient safety as well as to help the student make realistic plans to acquire the necessary knowledge and skill. Other students may choose safe assignments that do not challenge their abilities; the teacher's role is to support and encourage such students to take advantage of opportunities to achieve higher levels of knowledge and skill.

Skill Focus Versus Total Care Focus

As previously discussed, the traditional clinical assignment for nursing students is to give total care to one or more patients. However, not all learning objectives require students to practice total patient care. For example, if the objective is, "Assess patient and family preparation for postoperative recovery at home," the student does not have to provide total care to the postoperative patient to meet the objective. The student could meet the objective by interviewing the patient and family, reviewing the patient's records, and observing the patient's or family member's return demonstration of a dressing change. Additionally, total patient care is an integrative activity that can be accomplished effectively only when students are competent in performing the component skills.

All students do not need to be engaged in the same learning activities at the same time (Case & Oermann, 2004). Depending on their individual learning needs, some students might be engaged in activities that focus on developing a particular skill, while others could be practicing more integrative activities such as providing total patient care.

Student–Patient Ratio Options

Although the traditional clinical assignment takes the form of one student to one patient, there are other assignment options (Case & Oermann, 2004; Stokes & Kost, 2004). These options are described and compared as follows.

- *One student/one patient.* One student is responsible for certain aspects of care or for comprehensive care for one or more patients. The student works alone to plan, implement, and evaluate nursing care. This type of assignment is advantageous when the objective is to integrate many aspects of care after the student has learned the individual activities.
- *Multiple students/one patient.* Two or more students are assigned to plan, implement, and evaluate care for one patient. Each learner has a defined role, and all collaborate to meet the learning objective. Various models of dual or multiple assignment exist. For example, three students would read the patient record, review the relevant pathophysiology, and collaborate on an assessment and plan of care. Student A reviews information concerning the patient's medications, administers and documents all scheduled and p.r.n. medications, and manages the intravenous infusions. Student B focuses on providing and documenting all other aspects of patient care. Student C evaluates the effectiveness of the plan of care, assists with physical care when needed, interacts with the patient's family, and gives report to appropriate staff members. Members of the learning team can switch roles on subsequent days. This assignment strategy is particularly useful when patients have complex needs that are beyond the capability of one student, although it can be used in any setting with a large number of students and a low patient census. Other advantages include reducing student anxiety and teaching teamwork and collaborative learning.
- *Multiple students/patient aggregate.* A group of students is assigned to complete activities related to a community or population subgroup at risk for certain health problems. For example, a small group of students might be assigned to conduct a community assessment to identify an actual or potential health problem in the aggregate served by the clinical agency. Clinical activities would include interviewing community members and agency staff, identifying environmental and occupational health hazards, documenting the availability of social and health services, and performing selected physical assessments on a sample of the aggregate. The student group then would analyze the data and present a report to the

agency staff and community members. Advantages of this assignment strategy include promoting a focus on community as client, teaching collaboration with other health care providers and community members, and reinforcement of group process (Doerr et al., 1998)

Management Activities

Some clinical assignments are chosen to enable learners to meet outcomes related to nursing leadership, management and improvement of patient care, and meeting health care organizational goals. Undergraduate nursing students are usually introduced to concepts and skills of leadership and management in preparation for their future roles in complex health care systems. These students often benefit from clinical assignments that allow them to develop skill in planning and managing care for a group of patients. For example, a senior BSN student may enact the role of team leader for other nursing students who are assigned to provide total care for individual patients (Bradshaw, Rule, & Hooper, 2002). The student-as-team-leader may receive report about the group of patients from agency staff, plan assignments for the other students, give report to those students, supervise and coordinate work, and communicate patient information to staff members.

Master's and doctoral students may be preparing for management and administrative roles in health care organizations; their clinical activities might focus on enacting the roles of first-level or middle manager, patient care services administrator, or case manager. New staff nurse employees usually need to be oriented to the role of charge nurse; assignments to help them learn the necessary knowledge, skills, and attitudes should include practice in this role. Often, such clinical assignments involve the participation of a preceptor (see the discussion of models of teaching in Chapter 4, and Chapter 14, "Using Preceptors in Clinical Teaching").

Guided Observation

Observation is an important skill in nursing practice, and teachers should provide opportunities for learners to develop this skill systematically. Observing patients in order to collect data is a prerequisite to problem solving and clinical decision making. To make accurate and useful observations, the student must have knowledge of the phenomenon and the intellectual skill to observe it: the "what" and "how" of observation. As a clinical learning assignment, observation should not be combined with an assignment to provide care. If students do not have concurrent care responsibilities, they are free to choose the times and sometimes the locations of their observations. The focus should be on observing purposefully to meet a learning objective.

Observation also provides opportunities for students to learn through modeling. From observing another person performing a skill, the learner forms an image of how the behavior is to be performed, which serves as a guide to learning. For this reason, it is helpful to schedule learners to observe in a clinical setting before they are assigned to practice activities. However, scheduling an observation before the learner has acquired the prerequisite knowledge is unproductive; the student may not be able to make meaning out of what is observed.

Written observation guidelines can be used effectively to prepare learners for the activity and to guide their attention to important data during the observation itself. Table 7.1 is an example of an observation guide to prepare students for a

TABLE 7.1   Example of an Observation Guide

Operating Room Observation Guide

Purposes of the observation activity:

1. To gain an overview of perioperative nursing care in the intraoperative phase
2. To observe application of principles of surgical asepsis in the operating room
3. To distinguish among roles of various members of the surgical team

General information:

You are expected to prepare for this observation and to complete an observation guide while you are observing the surgical procedure. Please read your medical-surgical nursing textbook, pp. 195–200, for a general understanding of nursing roles in the intraoperative phase.

Bring this observation guide and a pen or pencil on the day of your observation. The guide will be collected and reviewed by the instructor at the end of the observation activity.

Most likely, you will observe either a coronary artery bypass graft or an aortic valve replacement. Please review the anatomy of the heart, specifically the coronary vessels and valves. In addition, read the following pages in your medical-surgical nursing textbook: coronary artery disease, pp. 1058–1059 and 1069–1085; valvular heart disease (aortic stenosis), pp. 1131–1132 and 1135–1139.

After you have completed your reading assignment, try to answer the questions in the first section of the observation guide ("Preparation of the Patient") related to preparations that take place before the patient comes to the operating room. Don't be afraid to make some educated guesses about the answers; we will discuss them and supply any missing information on the day of your observation.

Complete the remaining sections of the observation guide during your observation. The instructor will be available to guide the observation and to answer questions.

TABLE 7.1   (Continued)

Preparation of the Patient

A.   Who is responsible for obtaining the consent for the surgical procedure? Why?

B.   Who identifies the patient when he or she is brought into the operating room? Why?

C.   What other patient data should be reviewed by a nurse when the patient is brought to the operating room? Why?

D.   Who transfers the patient from transport bed to the operating room bed? What safety precautions are taken during this procedure?

E.   What is the nurse's role during anesthesia induction?

F.   When is the patient positioned for the surgical procedure? Who does this? What safety precautions are taken? What special equipment may be used?

G.   What is the purpose of the preoperative skin preparation of the operative site? When is it done? What safety precautions are taken?

H.   What is the purpose of draping the patient and equipment? What factors determine the type of drape material used? What safety precautions are taken? Who does the draping? Why?

I.   What nursing diagnoses are commonly identified for patients in the immediate preoperative and early intraoperative phases?

Preparation of Personnel

A.   Apparel: Who is wearing what? What factors determine the selection of apparel? How and when do personnel don and remove apparel items? What personal protective equipment is used and why?

(*continues*)

TABLE 7.1   Example of an Observation Guide (Continued)

B.   Hand antisepsis: Which personnel use hand antisepsis techniques to prepare for the procedure? When?

C.   Gowning and gloving: What roles do the scrub person and the circulator play?

Roles of Surgical Team Members

A.   Surgeons and assistants (surgical residents, interns, medical students)

B.   Nurses

C.   Anesthesia personnel

D.   Others (perfusion technologist, radiologic technologist, pathologist, etc.)

Maintenance of Aseptic Technique

A.   Movement of personnel

B.   Sterile areas/items

C.   Nonsterile areas/items

D.   Handling of sterile items

Equipment

A.   Lighting: Who positions it? How? When?

B.   Monitoring: What monitors are used? Who is responsible for setting up and watching this equipment?

C.   Blood/other fluid infusion: Who is responsible for setting up and monitoring this equipment?

TABLE 7.1   (Continued)

D.   Electrosurgical unit: What is this equipment used for? Who is responsible for it? What safety precautions are taken?

E.   Suction: What is this equipment used for? Who is responsible for setting up and monitoring it?

F.   Smoke evacuator: What is this equipment used for? Who is responsible for setting up and using it?

G.   Patient heating/cooling equipment: What is this equipment used for? Who is responsible for setting up and monitoring it?

H.   Other equipment:

Intraoperative and Early Postoperative Period Nursing Diagnoses

A.   What nursing diagnoses are likely to be identified for this patient in the intraoperative and early postoperative periods?

---

group observation activity in an operating room. Note the explicit expectations that students will read, think critically, and anticipate what they will see before the actual observation. The presence of an instructor or other resource person to answer questions and direct students' attention to pertinent items or activities is also helpful. Students may be asked to evaluate the observation activity by identifying learning outcomes, what they did and did not like about the activity, and the extent to which their preparation and the participation of the instructor was helpful. Table 7.2 is a sample evaluation tool for an observation activity.

Service-Learning

Another option for clinical learning assignments is service-learning. Service-learning differs from volunteer work, community service, fieldwork, and internships. Volunteer and community service focus primarily on the service that is

TABLE 7.2   Example of Student Evaluation of a Guided Observation Activity

---

Student Evaluation of OR Observation

1. To what extent did you prepare for this learning activity?
   - ____ 4. I completed all assigned readings and attempted answers to all questions on the first section of the observation guide.
   - ____ 3. I completed all assigned readings and attempted to answer some of the observation guide questions.
   - ____ 2. I completed some of the assigned readings and attempted to answer some of the observation guide questions.
   - ____ 1. I didn't do any reading but I tried to answer some of the observation guide questions before I came to the OR.
   - ____ 0. I didn't do any reading and I didn't answer any observation guide questions before I came to the OR.

2. How would you rate the overall value of this learning activity?
   - ____ 4. It was excellent; I learned a great deal.
   - ____ 3. It was very good; I learned more than I expected to.
   - ____ 2. It was good; I learned about as much as I expected to.
   - ____ 1. It was fair; I didn't learn as much as I expected to.
   - ____ 0. It was poor; I didn't learn anything of value.

3. How would you rate the value of the observation guide in helping you to prepare for and participate in the observation?
   - ____ 4. Extremely helpful in focusing my attention on significant aspects of perioperative nursing care.
   - ____ 3. Very helpful in guiding me to observe activities in the OR.
   - ____ 2. Helpful in guiding my observations, but at times distracted my attention from what I wanted to watch.
   - ____ 1. Only a little helpful; it seemed like a lot of work for little benefit.
   - ____ 0. Not at all helpful; it distracted me more than it helped me to observe what was going on in the OR.

4. How would you rate the helpfulness of the instructor who guided your OR observation?
   - ____ 4. Excellent; helped me to analyze, synthesize, and evaluate the activities I observed.
   - ____ 3. Very good; answered my questions and focused my attention on important activities.
   - ____ 2. Good; was able to answer some questions, attempted to make the activity meaningful to me.
   - ____ 1. Fair; I probably could have learned as much without an instructor present.
   - ____ 0. Poor; distracted me or interfered with my learning; I could have learned more without an instructor present.

TABLE 7.2   (Continued)

5. What was the most meaningful part of this learning activity for you? What was the most important or surprising thing you learned?

6. What was the least meaningful part of this observation activity? If there is something that you would change, suggest what would make it better.

provided to the recipients, and fieldwork and internships primarily focus on benefits to student learning. Service-learning intentionally combines the benefits to the community and to student learning in ways that are mutually satisfying (Sedlak, Doheny, Panthofer, & Anaya (2003). Service-learning is an academic credit-earning learning activity in which students

- participate in an organized service activity that meets identified community needs; and

- reflect on the service activity to gain a deeper understanding of course content, a broader appreciation of the discipline, and an enhanced sense of responsibility as a citizen (Bentley & Ellison, 2005).

Benefits of service-learning to students include developing skills in communication, critical thinking, and collaboration; developing a community perspective and commitment to health promotion in the community; awareness of diversity and cultural competence; and professional development and self-discovery (Bentley & Ellison, 2005; Sedlak et al., 2003). Benefits to the community arise from the first two of three principles of service-learning (Rodgers, 2001) that distinguish it from traditional clinical learning activities in nursing education:

1. The recipients of service control the service provided.

2. The recipients of service become better able to serve themselves and be served by their own actions.

3. Those who serve are learners who have significant control over what is learned.

The Pew Health Professions Commission 1993 report, *Health Professions Education for the Future: Schools in Service to the Community*, recommended that service-learning be incorporated into university nursing education to meet the increasing demand of community-based health care needs. As nursing education programs include more community-based learning activities, opportunities to incorporate service-learning increase. "Developing a community-based service learning experience requires the establishment of a relationship between the academic unit and the community to be served" (Rodgers, 2001, p. 244). For such partnerships to work effectively, there must be a good fit between the academic unit's mission and goals and the needs of the community (Rodgers).

As is true for any other clinical learning activity, planning for a service-learning activity begins with the teacher's decision that such learning activities would help students to achieve one or more course outcomes. The teacher should determine how many hours of clinical practice to allot to this activity, keeping in mind that the time spent in service-learning would replace and not add to the total time available for clinical activities for that course.

Before students participate in a service-learning activity, they should be required to prepare a learning contract that includes the following elements:

- The name of the community agency or group

- The clients or recipients of that agency's or group's services

- The services to be provided by the student

- A service objective related to a need that has been identified by the community or the community recipient of the proposed service

- A learning objective that is related to a course outcome, goal, or competency that the activity would help the student to achieve

Students may seek potential community groups and agencies in which they believe they could meet their learning needs, or the instructor may develop a list of such agencies and groups appropriate for a specific course from which students may choose a site. Examples of community settings and agencies that would be appropriate for service-learning include day-care centers, nursing homes, senior citizen centers, Meals on Wheels, the American Red Cross, Head Start, and a camp for children with disabilities, among many others (Bentley & Ellison, 2005; Rodgers, 2001; Sedlak et al, 2003).

Because service-learning is more than expecting students to use some of their clinical practice hours for service projects, faculty members should plan to spend as much time planning these activities as they do traditional clinical learning activities. Even though the teacher will not be with the students during the learning activity, the teacher must allow time to read and give feedback to students' reflective journal entries about their experiences or to participate in individual or group face-to-face reflective sessions. Faculty members may require students to do presentations of their service-learning projects, which the teachers themselves would observe and evaluate, another time requirement. And faculty members must also continue to interact with members of the community to evaluate the outcomes of service-learning from the perspective of the recipients of service and to continually nurture the partnerships that were established (Bentley & Ellison, 2005).

SUMMARY

This chapter presented a framework for selecting clinical learning assignments. Clinical teachers should select clinical assignments that are related to objectives, appropriate to students' levels of knowledge and skill, and challenging enough to motivate learning. Providing comprehensive nursing care to one or more patients is a typical clinical assignment, but it is not always the most appropriate choice.

Clinical teachers typically speak of "selecting patients" for clinical assignments. However, the primary role of the nursing student in the clinical area is that of learner, not nurse. Caring for patients is not synonymous with learning. Nursing students are *learning to care for* patients; they are not nurses with *responsibility for patient care*. In fact, early responsibility for patient care often creates anxiety that interferes with learning.

Factors affecting the selection of clinical assignments include the learning objectives of the clinical activity, needs of patients, availability and variety of learning opportunities in the clinical environment, and the needs, interests, and abilities of learners. The most important criterion for selection of clinical assignments usually is the learning objective. Each clinical activity should be an integral part of the course or educational program, and it is essential that the instructor, students, and staff members understand the goals of each clinical activity. Learning activities are selected and structured so that they relate logically and sequentially to the objective.

Individual learner characteristics such as educational level, previous experience, aptitude for learning, learning style, and specific needs, interests, and abilities should also influence the selection of clinical assignments. All learners do not have the same needs, so it is unreasonable to expect them to have the same learning assignments on any given day. Students who are able to achieve the objectives of the essential curriculum quickly might receive assignments from the enrichment curriculum that allow them to focus on their individual needs.

Patient needs and care requirements should also be considered when planning clinical assignments. The nursing care activities required by a patient may not present enough of a challenge to one learner or may be too complex for another. Patient wishes regarding student assignment should be respected. Nursing staff members who have provided care to these patients can often help the clinical teacher determine if student learning needs and specific patient and family needs both can be met through a particular clinical assignment.

Another factor affecting the selection of clinical assignments is the timing and availability of learning opportunities. Ideally, clinical learning activities are scheduled concurrently with relevant classroom content so that learners can apply knowledge to nursing practice immediately. The usual schedule of activities in the clinical facility may determine the optimum timing of learning activities. Some clinical settings are available both to patients and students only at certain times. In other settings, however, scheduling clinical learning assignments during evening or night hours or on weekends provides better opportunities to meet objectives.

Alternatives for making clinical assignments include selection by teacher or learner, focus on particular skills or integrative patient care, various student–patient ratio options, management activities, guided observation, and service-learning. Advantages and drawbacks of each alternative were discussed.

REFERENCES

Bentley, R., & Ellison, K. J. (2005). IMPACT of a service-learning project on nursing students. *Nursing Education Perspectives, 26,* 287–290.

Bradshaw, M. J., Rule, R., & Hooper, V. (2002). A joint junior-senior clinical experience. *Nurse Educator, 27,* 56–57.

Case, B., & Oermann, M. H. (2004). Teaching in a clinical setting. In L. Caputi & L. Engelmann (Eds.), *Teaching nursing: The art and science* (pp. 126–177). Glen Ellyn, IL: College of DuPage Press.

Doerr, B., Sheil, E., Baisch, M. J., Forbes, S., Howe, C J., Johnson, M., et al. (1998). Beyond community assessment into the real world of learning aggregate practice. *Nursing and Health Care Perspectives, 19,* 214–219.

Dunn, S. V., Stockhausen, L., Thornton, R., & Barnard, A. (1995). The relationship between clinical education format and selected student learning outcomes. *Journal of Nursing Education, 34,* 16–24.

Infante, M. S. (1985). *The clinical laboratory in nursing education* (2nd ed.). New York: Wiley.

Karuhije, H. F. (1997). Classroom and clinical teaching in nursing: Delineating differences. *Nursing Forum, 32,* 5–12.

Pew Health Professions Commission. (1993). *Health professions education for the future: Schools in service to the community.* San Francisco: UCSF Center for the Health Professions.

Rodgers, M. W. (2001). Service learning: Resource allocation. *Nurse Educator, 26,* 244–247.

Sedlak, C. A, Doheny, M., Panthofer, N., & Anaya, E. (2003). Critical thinking in students' service-learning experiences. *College Teaching, 51,* 99–103.

Stokes, L., & Kost, G. (2005). Teaching in the clinical setting. In D. M. Billings & J. A. Halstead, (Eds.), *Teaching in nursing: A guide for faculty* (2nd ed., pp. 325–348). St. Louis: Elsevier Saunders.

Chapter 8

Self-Directed Learning Activities

Some outcomes of clinical courses may be met by the students themselves through self-directed learning activities. These activities may involve instructional media such as videos on DVDs and CDs, computer-assisted instruction, virtual reality, Web-based methods, learning objects, independent study, and others. Faculty members have a wealth of instructional technologies to integrate into their clinical courses for students to acquire the prerequisite knowledge and skills, for review, and for learning new concepts and skills, among other uses.

There are many individual differences among nursing students that influence how they learn. Some students enter a clinical course with extensive knowledge and skills while others may lack the prerequisite behaviors for engaging in the learning activities. Differences in learning styles, preferences for teaching methods, cultural and ethnic backgrounds, and pace of learning all suggest a need for self-directed activities that reflect these individual variations among learners. With these activities, the responsibility for learning rests with the student.

There are varied types of self-directed activities for use in clinical teaching. Many of these activities are based on multimedia and instructional technology while others such as a literature review and critique may not incorporate media. Self-directed activities may be required for completion by all students to meet the outcomes of the clinical course or for use by individual students for reinforcement of learning, continued practice of skills, and remedial instruction. This chapter reviews self-directed learning activities appropriate for clinical teaching. The reader should recognize, however, that the activities involving multimedia are changing rapidly, and new technologies are continually being introduced for teaching and learning in clinical practice.

USING SELF-DIRECTED LEARNING ACTIVITIES

Self-directed learning activities are what the term suggests—activities directed by the students themselves. While planned by the teacher as part of the clinical activities, or recommended to meet specific learning needs, self-directed activities are intended for completion by the students on their own. These activities are typically self-contained units that students complete independently, often in a setting of their choice, and according to their own time frame. Computer-assisted instruction (CAI), for instance, may be completed in a computer or learning laboratory or at home at a time convenient for the student. The learner may move through the instruction at a fast or slow pace depending on the learning needs and may repeat content and activities until the competency is achieved. Many self-directed activities also include pre- and posttests for students to evaluate their own progress and learning at the end of the instruction.

Self-directed activities may be planned for completion by all students to meet certain clinical outcomes or by students on an individual basis to reflect their particular learning needs. For some clinical courses, all students may be required to complete self-directed activities as a means of acquiring essential knowledge for practice and developing course competencies. These activities, then, would be integrated in the clinical course during its development.

When students lack prerequisite knowledge and skills, or when remedial instruction is warranted for some students but not others, self-directed activities provide a means of meeting these learning needs without requiring all students to complete the same learning activities. In these instances, the self-directed activities assist individual students in gaining knowledge and skills they need for practice. Self-directed activities, therefore, are an important adjunct to clinical teaching.

Along with allowing students to learn in a setting of their choice and at a time convenient for them, self-directed activities encourage them to assume responsibility for their own learning, an important outcome of nursing programs. The student becomes a self-learner, seeking and using information for learning, rather than receiving it from the teacher (Hedberg, Brown, & Arrighi, 1997). As students progress through a nursing program, they may encounter outcomes that they are unable to meet because they lack the prerequisites for learning or need to review or practice their skills further. By identifying personal learning needs and seeking opportunities to meet them, students begin to develop skills they can use in the future when confronted with questions about nursing practice they are unable to answer and competencies they need to develop. Nursing programs provide the knowledge and competencies for entry into practice, but nurses need to be self-directed so they can keep current in their practice.

Although beneficial for students, self-directed learning requires their commitment and motivation. The teacher may plan strategies, such as periodic quizzes, to monitor student progress in completing the learning activities, provide feedback, and assist students in developing their self-discipline. In some courses faculty may establish time frames for completion of certain activities to better monitor progress and assure completion by the end of the clinical course.

Using Self-Directed Activities for Cognitive Skill Development

Self-directed activities that depict clinical situations and patient care scenarios are particularly effective for promoting problem-solving, decision-making, and critical-thinking skills. After viewing the clinical situation presented in media, in multimedia, or through other technologies, students may be asked to do any of the following:

- Identify the problems and issues to be solved and provide a supporting rationale

- Identify alternate problems that might be possible in the clinical situation

- Differentiate relevant and irrelevant information

- Develop careful and pointed questions to clarify the problems and issues further

- Identify additional data needed for decision making

- Identify multiple approaches for solving the clinical problems and issues they identified, alternate approaches possible, and advantages and disadvantages of each

- Compare varied decisions possible in a situation and outcomes

- Decide on the approach they would use, or decision they would make, and provide a rationale underlying their thinking

- Work backwards from the desired outcome to develop a plan for solving the problem (Nitko, 2004)

- Examine how key concepts and theories apply to the clinical situation depicted in the media or multimedia

- Analyze the clinical scenario using concepts and theories described in class, in readings, and through other learning activities as a way of transferring learning to clinical practice

- Identify assumptions made and how these influenced thinking

- Articulate different points of view (Oermann & Gaberson, 2006)

Using Self-Directed Activities for Value Development

Media and multimedia are also effective for teaching students professional nursing values and for students to examine their own beliefs and values that might influence their patient care. By viewing clinical situations depicted in media, students can gain awareness of other people's circumstances and their own values and beliefs. Students enter nursing programs with personal values and preset ideas that may influence their care and decisions they make in clinical practice. Analysis of scenarios shown in media provides a safe way for students to become more aware of their own value systems and beliefs. Through open-ended questions and a safe environment in which to discuss beliefs and feelings, students can begin to explore their own values and how they might affect decisions in clinical practice.

PLANNING SELF-DIRECTED ACTIVITIES

While self-directed activities are completed by students themselves, the teacher is responsible for planning those activities as part of the clinical course or recommending them for students to meet individual learning needs. Self-directed learning activities, similar to other types of clinical activities, should be consistent with the outcomes of the clinical course or competencies that students develop in that course. The main reason for their use in a course is their potential to assist students in achieving certain outcomes.

In planning self-directed activities, the teacher should consider the resources needed for their implementation. These resources include costs for developing materials, purchasing commercially available materials, and supporting software and hardware; equipment needed; space such as computer and other laboratories considering the numbers of students in the program; other requirements associated with using a particular technology; and resources needed by students. The time required for completion is another consideration in planning these activities for a course. The teacher should monitor the time that students take for each activity so this information is available for planning at a later time.

One way of ensuring effective planning and use of self-directed activities in a clinical course is to follow the acronym PLAN:

Plan activities that assist students in meeting the outcomes of the clinical course, individual learning needs, or both.

Link these activities with the resources of the nursing program and those needed by students.

Assess prerequisite knowledge and skills for initiating the self-directed activities, students' progress as they complete them, and learning outcomes.

Never assume that students will learn at the same rate and in the same way and instead allow for individualization in types of learning activities, rates of learning, and outcomes.

When incorporating self-directed activities in clinical courses, students should have directions as to specific activities to complete and due dates if required in the clinical course. It also is helpful to students to indicate how these particular activities promote achievement of the outcomes of the course and how they will be evaluated, if at all.

TYPES OF SELF-DIRECTED LEARNING ACTIVITIES

It is beyond the scope of this chapter to describe in detail all of the self-directed activities available for clinical teaching, particularly when considering the rapid growth of computer, Web-based, and other instructional technologies. While a number of self-directed methods are reviewed in this chapter, they do not represent an exhaustive list and instead present a sampling of these activities and how they might be used in clinical teaching. There are different ways of categorizing self-directed activities. In this chapter we group instructional media, such as videos on DVDs, CDs, and the Web; multimedia, including computer-assisted instruction, CD-ROMs, virtual reality, and the World Wide Web; learning objects; and independent study. The reader should also recognize that many of these methods use more than one technology; for instance, a computer simulation may include video, audio, and other multimedia.

Instructional Media

There are many types of media available for clinical teaching. Media are both print and nonprint, which provides an easy way of classifying media for use in clinical teaching (Table 8.1). Media include models; still visuals such as photographs, charts, posters, handouts, and slides; moving visuals such as videodiscs and DVDs; and audio media such as CDs and real audio (Zwirn, 2005).

Instructional media and multimedia promote learning through different senses, making it easier to comprehend difficult concepts and complex skills. Media that depict patient scenarios help students understand how concepts and theories are used in clinical practice and give them an idea of what a clinical situation is

TABLE 8.1   Types of Instructional Media

Print	Nonprint
Book	Audiotape
Brochure and pamphlet	CDs
Chart	CD-ROM
Handout, diagram, and other types of	Computer and related technology
written materials	DVDs
Poster	Film
Study guide	Model
Workbook	Overhead transparency
	Photograph
	Real audio
	Real object
	Slide
	Television
	Videodisc
	Videotape

like. This vicarious experience prepares learners for the reality of clinical practice. It also allows students to think critically in advance about a situation and possible decisions that could be made.

Another important use of media in clinical teaching is the ability to present clinical situations involving ethical dilemmas and value conflicts for students to analyze. When media are used in this way, students gain experience in analyzing and responding to an ethical dilemma before encountering it in actual practice. Media for this purpose also provide a means for students to examine their own values and beliefs that may influence care of patients and their interactions with staff and others in the practice setting.

Media are effective for showing clinical situations that would be inaccessible to students, close-up photographs, and procedures and technologies to be learned. With technological skills, media provide a way of demonstrating the use of equipment and how to carry out a procedure in the clinical setting, emphasizing critical elements of performance.

Multimedia

Multimedia include CAI, CD-ROM, virtual reality, World Wide Web, and many others. Multimedia are the combination of video, audio, text, and graphics that are often presented using computer technology (Zwirn, 2005). Multimedia, similar to media, may be used by all students to meet clinical learning outcomes or by individual students. A key concept of multimedia is the interaction between the computer program and learner. Many multimedia programs are interactive, providing feedback to students on their responses and engaging students actively in the learning process. Carty and Ong (2006) suggested that the most important characteristic of multimedia is their ability to deliver effective and flexible instruction that attracts learners' interest, keeps their attention, and accommodates different learning styles (p. 524).

Prior to using any multimedia for clinical teaching, the teacher should evaluate their content, including accuracy, organization, clarity in presenting the content, and comprehensiveness; relevance to the clinical course and clinical learning outcomes; usefulness for meeting individual student needs; currency in terms of clinical practice; extent of interaction between student and multimedia; cost; and resources needed for effective implementation (Table 8.2). One other aspect of this

TABLE 8.2   Evaluation of Multimedia for Clinical Teaching

Are the multimedia:

√ Relevant to the clinical course? Clinical learning outcomes? Clinical settings where students have practice?
√ Useful for meeting individual student needs?
√ Able to be modified or adapted to better meet the objectives and learner needs?
√ Of high technical quality (e.g., color, graphics, sounds, etc.)?

Is the content:

√ Accurate?
√ Organized logically?
√ Presented clearly?
√ Comprehensive?
√ In sufficient depth for clinical course and learners?
√ Up-to-date?

Does the instruction:

√ Provide for interaction with the student?
√ Give immediate feedback and reinforcement?
√ Maintain student interest?
√ Allow for entering and exiting the program as needed?
√ Adapt for individual student needs?

Is the cost worth the investment?

Are there sufficient resources for implementation?

evaluation relates to the appropriateness of the content for the clinical setting; with some multimedia, students may need to adapt interventions and procedures to their own clinical settings.

Computer-Assisted Instruction.   Computer-assisted instruction (CAI) uses the computer to guide learning; it provides instruction through interaction of the student and computer. There are many types of CAI programs for use in nursing education. Computer-assisted instruction may be used to present new content important for clinical practice, to promote application of concepts and theories to simulated clinical situations, as a review prior to clinical practice, and to provide remedial instruction for individual students. With some CAI, students can practice their problem solving and decision making in simulated scenarios. One main use of CAI is to guide students in applying concepts that they are learning in face-to-face and online courses to clinical situations and gaining experience in thinking through that situation before encountering it in clinical practice.

There are many CAI programs, and teachers need to be aware of what is available in their nursing education programs, clinical settings, or on the Web when they plan their courses. With this information faculty members can integrate CAI within their clinical courses and recommend specific programs to students when they need additional instruction or review. Often CAI programs incorporate questions for feedback to students, indicating which answers and decisions are correct or incorrect and why. The questions and answers also provide reinforcement for learning as students progress through the instruction. When not included with the CAI, faculty members can develop questions and answers for student self-assessment. Another advantage of CAI is that students can pace themselves through the instruction.

There are different types of CAI:

- *Drill-and-practice* CAI allows the student to practice previously learned content by asking questions about the content and having students respond to them. The CAI provides immediate feedback on the accuracy of these answers. Drill-and-practice CAIs are often used for teaching factual information such as definitions of medical terms and calculations of dosages of medications.
- *Tutorials* provide more feedback during the instruction than drill-and-practice CAI. Tutorials using branching techniques allow students to move forward to learn new content or backward if remedial instruction still is needed. For clinical teaching, tutorials may be used to present new content for practice or for remedial instruction.
- *Simulations* present a real-life situation for analysis and decision making. With a simulation, students make a series of clinical decisions similar to those needed in actual practice and receive immediate feedback on them. With some

simulations the learners' decisions influence subsequent information presented. Simulations are particularly appropriate for gaining practice in identifying data to collect, analyzing data in a simulated clinical situation, identifying problems and interventions, evaluating outcomes, and developing critical thinking and technological skills.

Computerized and interactive human patient simulators are being used increasingly in nursing education programs. These provide opportunity for students to develop knowledge and competencies for clinical practice, make clinical decisions in real time, develop technological skills not possible in many clinical settings, and achieve many other clinical outcomes (Jeffries, 2005, 2006; Jeffries, Hovancsek, & Clochesy, 2006; Seropian, 2003).

CD-ROM.   There are many CD-ROMs available for use in clinical teaching across all levels of nursing education. Some CD-ROMs teach skills such as measuring vital signs, administering medications, and inserting and discontinuing IVs. For example, *IV Therapy* CD-ROM teaches students about various delivery systems for IVs; uses video to show step-by-step how to start, maintain, and discontinue IVs; and explains complications of IV therapy and the nurse's role in preventing them. There are related case studies in which students need to think critically and make decisions about IV therapy (FITNE, 2005). Other CD-ROMs focus on care of patients with varied health problems.

With CD-ROMs faculty members can expose students to care of patients and clinical situations they may not have an opportunity to experience in the clinical setting. For example, not all students in a course may have a chance to care for a child with a critical illness or an adult patient with dialysis. By completing CD-ROMs on care of these patients, students can acquire essential knowledge, learn about typical interventions and why they are used in the patient's care, review related medication and treatments, and analyze related clinical scenarios. They can be completed by students independently, not taking in-class or online instruction time.

CD-ROMs can also be used in staff education. Smith and Lombardo (2005) described use of a CD-ROM to teach nurses about patient education. The CD-ROM has streaming video clips, audio, questions for critical thinking, case studies, and interactive practice activities. By using the CD-ROM nurses were able to complete the workshop on their own computers at a time convenient for them.

Virtual Reality.   In virtual reality, scenes that represent a real situation are displayed on a computer screen, and learners have an opportunity to actively participate in them. The components include a computer system with graphics linked to "an operator tactile feedback device" (Hammer & Souers, 2004, p. 151). Visualization on the computer screen simulates what the patient or procedure would look like in an actual clinical situation. Often the virtual reality system includes different software packages with scenarios to enhance students' learning and practice of skills. As students practice procedures, they receive audible feedback about their technique and decisions.

World Wide Web.   The World Wide Web (WWW) is a multimedia platform for accessing information that is organized in relationship to other information, enabling the student to retrieve it quickly and easily through different paths. The WWW gives learners access to large databases, enables them to find answers to questions about patient problems and clinical situations, and allows students to select pathways through this information that are appropriate for their own learning needs and interests. The Web provides access to a wealth of instructional resources that can be used in clinical teaching, such as, illustrations, photos, X-rays, and film clips, among others. When learning about a clinical concept, students can be directed to a Web site to view that concept.

The WWW relies on the use of hypertext, a multidimensional pathway linking words by associations (Gillham, 1998). A major advantage of hypertext for nursing education is that it allows for rapid navigation through large quantities of information (Gillham, 1998, p. 95). Given suitable computer and database access, students and nurses in practice can quickly retrieve information and gather possible answers to questions raised about patient care.

Many courses in nursing are now Web-based in which the entire course is online. McHugh (2006) advises faculty to make their Web courses multisensory and multidimensional, incorporating audio, visual, photos, animation, and other multimedia in them. The Web has opened many opportunities for self-directed activities to support clinical learning. Students may communicate with each other in the clinical group and with the teacher through e-mail, discussion boards, computer conferences, and chat rooms and may analyze cases and clinical issues in online discussions in small groups set up by the faculty member. Students may be directed to Web sites related to the clinical objectives or to explore specific clinical issues faced in their practice. In the beginning of a clinical course, for example, students may explore sites relevant to the area of clinical practice, such as oncology nursing, and evaluate each site for its usefulness in caring for these patients, in patient education, or for their own learning. If resources are available, self-directed activities on the Web are limited only by the teacher's creativity and willingness to explore new technologies.

Guidelines for Using Multimedia

With the wealth of multimedia available for clinical teaching, the teacher should first evaluate the quality and appropriateness of the multimedia for the intended learning outcomes. Not all multimedia are of high quality nor are they appropriate for the objectives or meeting learner needs. Here are other guidelines for using multimedia for clinical teaching:

- Prepare objectives to be achieved through completion of the multimedia.
- Consider assigning or recommending selected parts of a multimedia program that are most appropriate for the learning outcomes rather than the entire program.
- When parts of a multimedia program are used and when students complete multiple learning activities, provide written guidelines for them to follow that include the sequence for completing the activities. These guidelines, similar to a map, direct students through varied activities and segments of a program.
- Plan for some of the activities involving multimedia to be completed in pairs or small groups. Small group discussions about the content and possible answers to questions posed in the multimedia and the exchange of ideas about problems, approaches, and multiple ways of viewing clinical situations encourage problem solving, decision making, and critical thinking.
- Consider carefully the resources, hardware and software, needed for effective implementation of the multimedia. Programs completed in pairs and small groups often ease the burden for adequate hardware and software for the total number of students within the time limitations.
- Develop questions for students to answer as they progress through the multimedia and at the end of the instruction if feedback questions and a posttest are not already included. If the teacher intends for the multimedia to be used independently by students, then answers with a rationale should be included with the questions. The teacher should first review the multimedia program because many will have questions integrated throughout for student response. Questions also may be written to link the multimedia to the specific clinical objectives and help students relate the content to the clinical setting and types of clients for whom they are caring.
- Provide an opportunity for students to evaluate the multimedia in terms of quality, from a learner's perspective, and usefulness in developing knowledge and skills for clinical practice.

Learning Objects

Learning objects are small units of learning that are reusable, that is, one learning object may be used in different situations and courses and enhanced for more complex learning. With learning objects the goal is to divide the educational content into small bits or chunks of information that can be reused in different learning situations (Wiley, 2000). Beck (2005) indicates that learning objects typically take from 2 to 15 minutes to complete. Although learning objects are self-contained, and thus can be completed independently, they also can be grouped together into broader and more extensive collections of content.

Learning objects are developed to teach a single learning entity or concept (Wyatt & Royer, 2006). Many types of learning objects can be designed for use in clinical courses such as digital photographs of patients, conditions, procedures, and clinical situations; video clips and videos to teach clinical concepts; case studies for analysis with critical thinking questions; hyperlinks to Web pages and Internet resources; simulations; interactive games; and units of content taught with multimedia. For example, Baumann and DePablo (2005) developed a learning object on readability and patient education, which teaches strategies for creating readable educational documents for patients. Another example is a learning object in which students explore a virtual hospital wing, identify potential infection sources and risks, and design a plan to prevent infections (Bird & Bird, 2005).

Learning objects are valuable resources for use in distance education clinical courses and other Web-based courses. They can be stored in repositories or libraries of learning objects. Since they can be reused, faculty members can access these repositories as they are planning their clinical courses and can direct students to them to meet individual learning goals. MERLOT (Multimedia Educational Resource for Learning and Online Teaching) is a free resource for faculty and students (http://www.merlot.org/Home.po). It provides links to online learning objects with peer reviews and assignments.

Independent Study

Independent study allows the student freedom in deciding on his or her own learning goals, strategies for learning, and how the learning outcomes will be evaluated as part of the clinical course. The teacher and student typically collaborate on the objectives to be met through independent study so they relate to the clinical goals and are reasonable within the time frame. A contract may be established between the teacher and student outlining the goals to be met through the independent study project, types of learning activities to be completed, evaluation methods and products of learning to be submitted as part of the clinical course, and dates for completion of these. Independent study is particularly useful when students want to explore a new area of clinical practice or a patient problem and interventions in depth.

SUMMARY

Many clinical objectives and competencies may be met by the students themselves through self-directed learning activities. Whether planned by the teacher as part of the clinical activities or recommended to meet specific learning needs, self-directed activities are intended for completion by the students on their own. These activities are typically self-contained units that students complete independently, often in a setting of their choice, and according to their own time frame. Self-directed activities encourage students to assume responsibility for their own learning, an important outcome of nursing programs.

Self-directed activities may be completed by all students to meet certain clinical competencies or by students on an individual basis to reflect their particular learning needs. Similar to other types of learning activities, they should be consistent with the outcomes of the clinical course.

In planning self-directed activities, the teacher should consider the resources needed for their implementation. These resources include costs for developing materials, purchasing commercially available materials, and supporting software and hardware; equipment needed; space such as computer laboratory space; other requirements associated with a particular technology; and resources needed by students. The time required for completion is another consideration in planning these activities for a course.

Self-directed activities are categorized as instructional media, such as videos; multimedia including computer-assisted instruction, CD-ROM, virtual reality, and the World Wide Web; learning objects; and independent study. Instructional media and multimedia promote learning through different senses, making it easier to comprehend difficult concepts. Media and multimedia that depict patient care scenarios help students understand how concepts and theories are used in practice and give them an idea of what a clinical situation is like. This vicarious experience prepares learners for the reality of clinical practice.

Multimedia are the combination of video, audio, text, and graphics that are presented using computer technology. Multimedia for use in clinical teaching are extensive; it is up to the teacher to be creative and willing to integrate these new technologies into clinical courses.

REFERENCES

Baumann, L., & DePablo, M. (2005). *Readability and patient education.* Retrieved February 5, 2006, from http://neatproject.org/learning_objects/read.htm#

Beck, R. J. (2005, June 3). *Learning objects: What?* Retrieved February 5, 2006, from http://www.uwm.edu/Dept/CIE/AOP/LO_what.html

Bird, P., & Bird, D. (2005). *Preventing hospital acquired infection.* Retrieved February 5, 2006, from http://neatproject.org/learning_objects/hospital_infections.htm

Carty, B., & Ong, I. (2006). The nursing curriculum in the information age. In V. K. Saba & K. A. McCormick (Eds.), *Essentials of nursing informatics* (4th ed., pp. 517–532). New York: McGraw-Hill.

FITNE Inc. (2005). *IV Therapy.* Retrieved February 5, 2006, from http://www.fitne.net/ivtherapy.htm

Gillham, D. (1998). Using hypertext to facilitate nurse education. *Computers in Nursing, 16*, 95–98.

Hammer, J., & Souers, C. (2004). Infusion therapy: A multifaceted approach to teaching in nursing. *Journal of Infusion Nursing, 27*, 151–156.

Hedberg, J., Brown, C., & Arrighi, M. (1997). Interactive multimedia and web-based learning: Similarities and differences. In B. H. Khan (Ed.), *Web-based instruction* (pp. 47–58). Englewood Cliffs, NJ: Educational Technology Publications.

Jeffries, P. R. (2005). A framework for designing, implementing, and evaluating simulations in nursing. *Nursing Education Perspectives, 26*, 28–35.

Jeffries, P. R. (2006). Designing simulations for nursing education. In M. H. Oermann & K. T. Heinrich (Eds.), *Annual review of nursing education* (Vol. 4, pp. 161–177). New York: Springer Publishing.

Jeffries, P. R., Hovancsek M. T., & Clochesy, J. M. (2006). Using clinical simulation in distance education. In J. M. Novotny & R. H. Davis (Eds.), *Distance education in nursing* (2nd ed., pp. 83–99). New York: Springer Publishing.

McHugh, M. (2006). Teaching a Web-based course: Lessons from the front. In J. M. Novotny & R. H. Davis (Eds.), *Distance education in nursing* (2nd ed., pp. 15–45). New York: Springer Publishing.

Nitko, A. J. (2004). *Educational assessment of students* (4th ed.). Upper Saddle River, NJ: Pearson Prentice Hall.

Oermann, M. H., & Gaberson, K. B. (2006). *Evaluation and testing in nursing education* (2nd ed.). New York: Springer Publishing.

Seropian, M. (2003). General concepts in full scale simulation: Getting started. *Anesthesiology Analog, 97*, 1695–1705.

Smith, J. A., & Lombardo, N. (2005). Patient education workshop on CD-ROM: An innovative approach for staff education. *Journal for Nurses in Staff Development, 21*, 43–46.

Wiley, D. A. (2000). Connecting learning objects to instructional design theory: A definition, a metaphor, and a taxonomy. In D. A. Wiley (Ed.), *The instructional use of learning objects: Online version*. Retrieved February 5, 2006, from http://reusability.org/read/chapters/wiley.doc

Wyatt, T. H., & Royer, L. (2006). Using learning objectives to enhance distance education. In J. M. Novotny & R. H. Davis (Eds.), *Distance education in nursing* (2nd ed., pp. 101–112). New York: Springer Publishing.

Zwirn, E. E. (2005). Using media, multimedia, and teachnology-rich learning environments. In D. M. Billings & J. A. Halstead (Eds.), *Teaching in nursing: A guide for faculty* (2nd ed., pp. 377–396). St. Louis: Elsevier Saunders.

Chapter 9

Clinical Simulation

Suzanne Hetzel Campbell

Clinical simulation is rapidly earning a place in nursing education as a viable option to supplement clinical practice with live patients. Simulation will never replace actual student contact with real patients, but it will make student and faculty time in actual clinical settings more valuable and cost-effective. The growing nursing shortage has stimulated an interest in nursing as a career and more applications to nursing education programs, but numbers of nursing faculty members are not increasing at the same pace, creating capacity limits in classrooms and clinical settings. In addition, the health care environment has grown in complexity with an increased use of technology and higher acuity levels of patients who are older, frailer, and have more comorbidity. Finally, specialty clinical areas such as obstetrics, pediatrics, and intensive care units often limit nursing student activities to observation rather than hands-on patient care and greatly restrict the number of students placed on those units. Nursing faculty members are challenged to prepare students for this complex environment where they must think critically, act quickly, and communicate effectively with their multidisciplinary team members. Long orientation programs for new nurses are a thing of the past, and nursing and health care administrators expect competent new graduates who quickly function independently (Morton, 1997). This chapter discusses clinical simulation as a valuable tool in the clinical education of nursing students.

BACKGROUND

Simulations, as defined in a National Council of State Boards of Nursing (NCSBN) position statement (2005), are "activities that mimic reality of a clinical environment and are designed to demonstrate procedures, decision-making and critical thinking through techniques such as role-playing and the use of devices such as interactive videos or mannequins" (see also Jeffries, 2005). Simulation allows faculty members to take substance-specific information, such as a client's personal characteristics, health information, family components, and physical, mental, and emotional state, and weave it into a real-life scenario that enhances a student's comprehension of the material because it is meaningful (Hertel & Millis, 2002). In the case of clinical nursing scenarios, simulation provides an opportunity to suspend belief of what is "real" to produce a risk-free, hands-on opportunity to practice a clinical situation involving patient monitoring, management, communication, and multidisciplinary collaboration. Simulation activities can enhance learning, critical thinking, and practice in specific areas for individuals in a variety of professions.

The earliest uses of simulation in the health care field were primarily in medical education, including medical schools, emergency room training, anesthesia crisis management, residents in trauma rotations, and even first responders for cardiac care (Bond, Kostenbader, & McCarthy, 2001; Cooper et al., 2000; Freeman et al., 2001; Gaba, Howard, & Fish, 2001; Kurrek & Fish, 1996; Marshall et al., 2001; Morgan, Cleave-Hogg, McIlroy, & Devitt, 2002). In nursing, simulation has been used to teach clinical decision making, critical care, and cardiopulmonary resuscitation (Collins, Edwards, & Graves, 2006; Hamilton, 2005; Henneman & Cunningham, 2005; Hjelm-Karlsson & Stenbeck, 1997; Kappus, Leon, Lyons, Meehan, & Hamilton-Bruno, 2006; Long, 2005). The use of human patient simulators (HPS), such as Laerdal/Medical's SimMan®, has increased due to the decreasing cost of the equipment and software and the acceptance of this teaching method (Seropian, Brown, Gavilanes, & Driggers, 2004b). Using simulation-based pedagogy allows students to integrate psychomotor, critical thinking, and communication skills and gain self-efficacy prior to entering the clinical setting (Babenko-Mould, Andrusyszyn, & Goldenberg, 2004; Goldenberg, Andrusyszyn, & Iwasiw, 2005; Madorin & Iwasiw, 1999; Rhodes & Curran, 2005; Schumacher, 2004). There is an opportunity for evaluation and assessment of student skills with options for remediation and continued learning. The active learning component of simulation adds to the variety of learning styles that today's students require to maintain engagement in the learning process and to retain the material learned.

Finally, the Commission on Collegiate Nursing Education (CCNE) accreditation standards encourage the use of innovative teaching methods and the introduction of technology and informatics to improve student learning (CCNE, 2003). In addition, the NCSBN emphasized the need for nursing student clinical experiences with real patients but acknowledged the value of clinical simulation, under the guidance of qualified faculty members who can provide feedback and facilitate reflection, in complementing actual patient contact. The Institute of

Medicine's report, *To Err is Human: Building a Safer Health System*, raised public awareness of the need to increase patient safety (Kohn, Corrigan, & Donaldson, 2000). Simulation is an innovative teaching method that uses technology and informatics, involves faculty guidance and feedback, and increases the competency of nursing students and practicing nurses to provide safe patient care.

TYPES OF SIMULATION

There are different levels of simulation, as well as a variety of types of simulation. The levels of simulation include low fidelity (less precise reproductions), such as a disembodied pelvis for catheter insertion simulation or foam arm for intramuscular injection simulation, sometimes referred to as "task-trainers." Moderate-fidelity simulators provide some feedback to the student, such as heart and lung sounds, and work well when introducing students to beginning skills. The Vital-Sim® (Laerdal/Medical) is an example that allows practice of vital signs and physical assessment techniques. Finally, high-fidelity simulators are those that produce the most lifelike scenarios, reacting to student manipulations in realistic ways, such as speaking, coughing, and demonstrating chest movements and pulses. High-fidelity HPSs, such as SimMan® (Laerdal/Medical), respond to pharmacological and physical manipulations, either manually or by preprogrammed software (Seropian et al., 2004b). The computer logs and potential for video-recording interactions between students and HPSs provide concrete feedback for student learning, assessment, and evaluation.

The types of simulation can vary from the high-fidelity HPS models to computer-assisted instruction that allows for live interaction with a simulated patient and decision making regarding care. These programs provide feedback to help students learn about the accuracy of their thinking and actions. Examples of these computer-assisted simulations include SimHosp®, SimClinic®, and Virtual IV® (Engum & Jeffries, 2003). Another tool is the Visible Human Dissector (VHD), which provides three-dimensional visualizations of photographic anatomy from the Visible Human Project® that allow for a variety of views and approaches to the study of anatomy (www.toltech.net).

There are Web technologies, with many programs developed for nursing instruction, from auscultation of heart and lung sounds to infant Apgar scoring. The availability of these technologies varies; some are presently free on the World Wide Web (such as the Wisconsin Online Resource Center, http://www.wisc-online.com/), others are bundled with textbook and workbook purchases, and some software can be purchased. These technologies can be incorporated into a hybrid course online, used in the classroom prior to a case study, or assigned in preparation for a simulation experience. The plethora of materials requires nurse educators to keep up with what is available to supplement planned clinical simulation activities.

Finally, the value of electronic medical record (EMR) use to patient safety and staff efficiency, as well as the role of the nurse in EMR use, has been documented (Valentine, 2005; Weir, Hoffman, Nebeker, & Hurdle, 2005). Some nursing programs are experimenting with the use of EMRs as a teaching tool to enhance clinical simulation. Individual communities or records have been created by faculty members using university or medical center resources; these scenarios provide students much in-depth information that adds to the feeling of reality. Students also gain practice navigating the software systems and learn to record their findings in this efficient and effective way (Donahue & Thiede, 2006; Eichenwald, 2004; Sheets, 2006).

DECIDING TO USE SIMULATION AS A TEACHING STRATEGY

Advantages and Implications

Several advantages of simulation-focused pedagogy have already been described. The decreased anxiety and increased self-confidence of students reported in some of the studies helps them to interact more comfortably with patients when they are in actual clinical settings. The opportunity to practice teamwork as students role-play helps them to take ownership for their role and enhances critical thinking skills, clinical performance, and competence. These benefits should result in shorter orientation periods in the transition from student to employee, but verification with empirical data is not yet available.

Other advantages include a controlled environment with reproducible and predictable results, especially if using a high-fidelity HPS with software. Once students and faculty members become familiar with the technology, it is easy to use, and it allows several students to experience the scenario in different ways at once. Some students find it to be less stressful than actual clinical activities, and it also provides an engaging, even entertaining learning activity (Seropian et al., 2004b).

Disadvantages and Challenges

Although simulation provides rich learning opportunities, it also presents challenges. Foremost are financial constraints when simulation involves purchasing the equipment and renovating buildings to accommodate the technology so that the scenarios can be run in a convenient and timely manner. There is added expense for maintenance of equipment and consumables as well. If minimal renovations are required, the process may proceed more smoothly, and many programs are making do with their available space. In addition, nursing programs are finding unique ways to raise funds for new labs and equipment, including grants, advisory boards, and partnerships (Appel, Campbell, Lynch, & Novotny, 2006). However, a vision of simulation-focused pedagogy, with the inherent tools available, is necessary for a meaningful and successful simulation program (Seropian, Brown, Gavilanes, & Driggers, 2004a; Seropian et al., 2004b). Other challenges include a faculty and staff learning curve involved in the development of a curriculum that incorporates simulation-focused pedagogy and in the smooth operation of the technology. There is an assumption of a certain level of computer literacy among the faculty and students to use the variety of simulation techniques discussed in this chapter. Therefore, simulation-focused curriculum requires more faculty, staff, and student development and training, as well as more time.

Educational Practices

A variety of educational practices are useful when incorporating simulation into a nursing education program. By engaging learners directly in the simulation, active learning occurs. Providing constructive feedback during the debriefing session, allowing students to view a DVD recording of their performance, or getting suggestions and critiques from classmates who may be viewing them in a nearby classroom all allow feedback for enhanced student performance (Henneman & Cunningham, 2005; Hravnak, Tuite, & Baldisseri, 2005; Johnson-Russell & Anderson, 2006). Because students learn through many different styles, simulation allows the incorporation of different teaching strategies.

Ideally, students have an assignment prior to the simulation—including but not limited to, reading, viewing a videotape, DVD, or online presentation (possibly via pod-casting)—and computer-assisted instruction. The simulation may begin with a few minutes of didactic information provided to a group of students in the classroom setting. Perhaps the teacher uses a scenario from SimHosp® to prepare the students for similar critical thinking and actions that they will face in the simulation. Dividing the class into teams enhances competitiveness and desire to do well. Each group of students then learns the background of a patient (the HPS) and other information that they need to enact the scenario, and they are assigned roles. The teacher, ideally controlling the simulation from a separate room, is able to use a preprogrammed scenario that incorporates verbal replies from the HPS and changes in vital signs that reflect student actions, and records all events of the scenarios.

This variety of teaching styles—auditory, kinesthetic, visual, olfactory, and emotionally experiential—assists learners to apply knowledge in a way that didactic methods fail. The simulation incorporates the teacher's presence, but during the actual time spent working with the HPS, teachers allow students to make mistakes and find their own way. Specific time frames for introduction of the scenario and preparation for it, actual running of the simulation, and debriefing must be carefully calculated ahead of time. Actual time-on-task should not vary greatly between students. Opportunities for collaboration are present in the preparatory period when students work together in groups and in role-playing during the scenario in which each student has a different part to play, and learning continues as students review and critique their own and other students' learning. Some students report that although they are uncomfortable enacting a scenario, they understand the value of peer observation and shared learning opportunity (Russell & Campbell, 2006).

Implementing Simulation

The implementation of simulation depends on the level of complexity, the level of technology, and the specific use for individual courses. The beginning user may learn lung and heart sounds by performing assessments on a moderate-fidelity simulator. Beginning use of simulation may thus occur for the teaching of psychomotor skills in a health assessment or clinical techniques course (Ham & O'Rourke, 2004). Students were found to have reduced anxiety with peer instruction in the learning laboratory (Owens & Walden, 2001); this effect is worthy of study with simulations as well.

An intermediate user in a medical-surgical or specialty course would be better prepared to use simulation for patient care involving less complex procedures, such as the management of pain or other common symptoms (e.g., urinary tract infection symptoms) (McCausland, Curran, & Cataldi, 2004). The advanced user might be incorporating intensive care and critical physiology simulations, such as severe asthma attack, ventilator assessment, or cardiac arrest (Henneman & Cunningham, 2005). In addition, advanced users might be studying specialty areas and populations using VitalSim® (Laerdal/Medical) or SimBaby® (Laerdal/Medical) for obstetric and pediatric experiences (Clinton, 2006; Goetz & Nissen, 2005; McCartney, 2005; Ravert, 2006; Yaeger et al., 2004). For teaching care of a population as client, simulation has been used for mass casualty incident training (Kobayashi, Shapiro, Suner, & Williams, 2003). This type of training could be modified for two levels of students—early in the program during a health care delivery system course, focusing on specific aspects of that system, and then later in the program as part of public health and leadership courses, in which expectations of student performance would include triaging and taking on a leadership role.

The level of technology used in clinical simulation depends on several factors, namely, faculty comfort, the technology available, and support for the use of technology. Nursing education programs that have access to information technology (IT) support, ideally designated IT staff members to support the program, are making the most progress with incorporating simulation smoothly into their programs. In addition, university services that support academic excellence with resources and specialists can assist with faculty development, and other departments can help incorporate components that will make the simulation feel more real. For example, faculty members in a university department of communication may be able to assist nursing faculty members with the dialogue component of scenarios. Performing arts faculty members and students can add to the contextual experience by role-playing distraught family members; nursing faculty members might apply some of their rich clinical experience by playing a spouse, parent, or child of the HPS. The more assistance nurse educators receive with the planning and implementation of the scenarios, the better the learning experience for teachers and students alike. A key factor to the level of technology used is to start simple and then increase complexity. Many nursing education programs have started by running a few simple scenarios "on the fly" (not using preprogrammed software) and have found that increasing complexity in small increments was not as hard as initially feared.

Once a nursing education program has embraced simulation-focused pedagogy, the next question is where to use simulation in the courses and in the curriculum. As faculty members outline the type of material to be covered, they can better determine where and when it should be placed in the course. Deciding whether the simulation will be introductory material or supplementary to class is up to individual teachers. Using a curriculum grid to outline courses, examining threads, content, and key areas of importance, will allow for a coordinated mapping of potential simulation activities. Seeing what scenarios are already available (e.g., downloadable from a Web site such as the Laerdal Patient Simulator User Site at http://www.laerdal.com/document.asp?docID=1264506) and building on those, as well as working in collaboration with other nursing education programs or clinical sites will assist with the planning and implementation phase (Berryman, Armstrong, & Zenoni, 2006). The ideal is to provide the faculty with release time to refurbish courses within a simulation-focused pedagogy, including scenario development and implementation.

GETTING STARTED CREATING SCENARIOS

Some basic ways to begin creating scenarios involve examining the institutional and nursing program mission statement, philosophy, and curricular objectives. When creating scenario objectives and guided reflection questions, the program, course, and unit objectives can be used as guidelines. It is important to identify essential learning outcomes, taking into consideration social and demographic trends specific to the geographic area and incorporating cultural sensitivity, spirituality, and ethical considerations. The level of the students, specific course objectives, and faculty personal clinical expertise all need to be considered when specifying an appropriate learning outcome. Other suggestions for creating scenarios include reviewing course evaluations, licensure and certification exam results by subject area, communication with clinical facilities, and other program evaluation data to identify essential learning needs of students (Chambers, 2006).

It is important to involve all faculty members in scenario writing, making content experts responsible for specific scenarios. Developing a template or blueprint for teachers to use as they develop scenarios will increase consistency as well as encourage them to start with basic information (e.g., identifying three to five simulation objectives and learning outcomes). It helps to have a champion who empowers faculty colleagues to create lively and interesting scenarios. Providing resources including support, props, time to practice, and space and time for the development of scenarios will further encourage full participation. Reviewing scenarios for accuracy, current evidence-based practice guidelines, and unnecessary distracters will ensure the quality of the simulation experience for all (Chambers, 2006).

Once a scenario has been written using the template, it is time to transfer it to the simulator. There are two options for running the simulator: manually, or "on the fly," and by automatic preprogramming. The manual mode allows flexibility and minimal time investment in advance because no prewritten programs are required, but it requires a talented and dynamic instructor with content expertise who responds quickly to student interventions. The automatic mode is more rigid and needs a knowledgeable individual to write the program, requiring considerable time investment in advance of implementation. The preprogrammed version allows the simulator to automatically respond to student interventions and produces clear event menus that can be standardized for evaluation and research. Lastly, the automatic mode results in the creation of valuable scenarios that can be used consistently over time. A scenario, once created in a preprogrammed mode, can be modified to meet the needs of students at various levels and at various times throughout the program. In addition, objectives and distracters can be added, settings can be changed, and roles can be altered to create new and more complex scenarios from simpler ones (Chambers, 2006). Simulation templates usually include five characteristics: objectives, fidelity, complexity, cues, and debriefing and guided reflection.

Objectives

The first characteristic, objectives, reflects the desired learning outcomes of the simulation. Objectives can focus on key areas such as safety, basic assessment skills, problem-focused assessment, intervention, delegation, and communication. As part of the template these objectives may be clearly identified as psychomotor skills and cognitive skills, and a list of skills to review prior to the simulation may be provided to students (Chambers, 2006).

Fidelity

The fidelity characteristic relates to the setting or environment (e.g., type of unit, institution, or home). The simulation provides a realistic environment by specifying the necessary simulator or manikin needed, the recommended mode for the simulation with rationale (e.g., microphone for communication), roles of participants and guidelines for each role, information about the patient, and any necessary props, including but not limited to

- equipment attached to the manikin (e.g., IV, catheter, oxygen);
- equipment available in the room (e.g., IV pump, emergency cart);
- medications and fluids;
- diagnostic test results (e.g., laboratory tests, X-rays);
- documentation forms (e.g., admission order, medication orders, flow sheet, EMR);
- other props (e.g., clothing, wig, eyeglasses for the HPS).

The written report on the HPS also will be created under this characteristic. Any references used, such as evidenced-based practice guidelines, protocols, or algorithms should cite the author, year, and page (Chambers, 2006). For use in undergraduate nursing programs, the National Council Licensure Examination test plan categories also can be used to focus the fidelity of a simulation as well. These categories include

- safe, effective care environment, both the management of care and safety and infection control;
- health promotion and maintenance;
- psychosocial integrity;
- physiologic integrity, including basic care and comfort, pharmacological and parenteral therapies, reduction of risk potential, and physiologic adaptation (Chambers, 2006).

Complexity

The complexity characteristic allows for adapting the developed scenarios to different levels and building from simple to complex. Some suggestions for changing the complexity include the following:

- Introduce a family member who is hard to handle.

- Have the patient be cared for directly in the ER to allow for NG tube and IV insertions.

- Develop an issue related to cultural or religious affiliation, such as requesting a spiritual support person or asking for ethnic foods.

- Provide opportunities for delegation or leadership (e.g., team leader for a resuscitation scenario).

Cues

The cues characteristic is reflective of the HPS's capability to replicate humanistic functions (e.g., cardiovascular, respiratory, and vocal responses) and to react to external stimuli (Jones, 2002). For example, within the first 2 minutes of the start of the scenario, if the student does not introduce himself or herself to the patient, the HPS will ask, "Who are you?" (Chambers, 2006). As the scenario plays out, if the student offers a drink or ice chips to a patient with NPO status, the HPS will mention, "My last nurse would not let me have water!" If the student does not explain rationale for the antibiotic, the HPS will ask nervously, "What are you giving me?" Finally, if the student attempts to give morphine sulfate for pain as ordered, failing to recognize the patient's allergy, the HPS will state angrily, "What is that??? You know I'm allergic to morphine, don't you?" These cues can be directly programmed into the scenario or run by the controller as the scenario unfolds. In a real clinical situation the patient may or may not react similarly and these responses add to the level of realism of the simulation, enhancing the student's learning.

Debriefing and Guided Reflection

The fifth characteristic involves debriefing and providing an opportunity for guided reflection of the simulation. This characteristic has been identified as crucial for students' learning and satisfaction with their simulation experience.

Adequate time must be arranged to provide sufficient debriefing. Identifying important concepts or curricular outcomes will help in planning the questions for debriefing; once again, a general template will allow consistency among students and faculty alike. Objectives for debriefing include answering student questions to help them clarify their thinking, release any emotional tension, and link the simulation to real life while reinforcing specific teaching points (Fritzsche, Leonard, Boscia, & Anderson, 2004). The instructor's role during debriefing is that of facilitator rather than evaluator. Prior to debriefing, the teacher should review the objectives of the simulation and discuss confidentiality as well as teacher expectations of students' participation in evaluating themselves and their group members (Haskvitz & Koop, 2004). Initial questions to guide reflection may focus on

- students' primary concerns in the scenario;
- anything they missed on report;
- assessment of their knowledge and skill capabilities to manage the situation, and areas requiring further practice;
- what went well;
- what they would do differently the next time;
- how the group performed (Chambers, 2006).

Additional questions might probe further into specifics about students' familiarity with the patient's condition, the environment, the techniques, interventions, or medications used during the scenario. Asking students to identify content that helped them succeed in the scenario and where they received it from (classroom, computer-assisted instruction, presentations, scenario preparation) will guide the teacher to improve the scenario. Having students examine communication and team collaboration, as well as their own reactions, emotions, and professional behavior during the scenario, will help them to critically assess their performance (Johnson-Russell & Anderson, 2006).

Finally, some closing statements about what students identified as going well, areas they need to work on, areas of improvement, and take-home points will help to summarize the experience. Thanking students for their participation and stating the teacher's appreciation of their attention, efforts in enacting the scenario, and sharing their reflections provides positive reinforcement. Using anonymous surveys for evaluation will also provide important information for future simulation development and performance (Johnson-Russell & Anderson, 2006).

SETTING UP A SIMULATION CENTER

Interest in creating simulation centers in nursing education programs and health care settings is increasing rapidly. The stimulus for the creation of some simulation centers is a directed donation for the purchase of an HPS, resulting in the development of a plan to create a center where students can learn in a risk-free, hands-on environment. With the increasing affordability of HPSs and software, and the growing number and value of grants and donations available for the education of nurses, it is an ideal time to plan a simulation lab, regardless of the size of the nursing education program.

Identify who will use the lab (students, undergraduate or graduate; staff nurses; other health care professionals) and what the labs will be used for prior to creating a concrete plan. If the lab is basically for the education of undergraduate and graduate student nurses, then acquiring grants to renovate the building and the equipment necessary to run simulations will be the priority, working with faculty and administrators to plan for the staff support to keep it running when the grants are gone. Partnerships between a nursing education program and various health care facilities to allow orientation, training, and continuing staff development for their employees in the new simulation center offer a potential source of income to sustain the operation of the center. The use of simulation labs may be offered to relevant government and community disaster response organizations and groups for practice of emergency preparedness, either for a fee or as an in-kind donation. Universities that use simulation labs for evaluation and research can often provide graduate students to assist with running scenarios and collecting data (Larew, Lessans, Spunt, Foster, & Covington, 2006). Some software publishers allow use of their EMR systems for product testing (Eichenwald, 2004). Other manufacturers of medical equipment such as pumps, ventilators, and medication dispensing systems may provide prototypes of their equipment for testing in the simulation lab.

There are wide variations in the quantity and type of simulation space. The scenarios described earlier in this chapter implied the use of a control room with a mirrored view into the scenario rooms and technology to deliver video images of the scenario live into a classroom for observation and interaction with peers. Specialty labs may include an anesthesia and operating room with working ventilator, especially for those academic centers with graduate programs that prepare Certified Registered Nurse Anesthetists. Some specialty labs may be set up to convert easily between emergency department, intensive care, and acute care hospital room environments. Having separate rooms for medium-fidelity simulation practice and specialty care such as obstetrics (with a birthing bed) and neonatal intensive care (incubators with infant HPSs) will add to the number of students that can be accommodated as well as the variety of experiences they can have. In addition, a home care lab is ideal for practicing problem-solving situations unique to this setting such as patient transfer within a standard size home bathroom and assessment of the home environment.

Nursing education programs affiliated with academic health centers may have standardized patients available to them (especially for pelvic, breast, and prostate exams). Practice with standardized patients can be invaluable learning opportunities for students, especially nurse practitioners. However, for students who do not have this option available, well-planned simulation experiences can meet their needs.

Nursing faculty members need to work closely with university administrators and facilities managers to resolve space and design issues in the development of the plan. Touring other simulation labs, seeking advice from HPS vendors, and learning about the design of other labs through virtual tours on the Internet or during conference sessions are ways to gather ideas and gain inspiration. Beyond development of the space itself, specific policies and procedures related to the simulation lab need to be put into place. Some policies surrounding authorization for taping of students and confidentiality issues need to be developed. Additionally, ground rules for professional behavior and attire will enhance the realness of the experience.

EVALUATING SIMULATIONS

Evaluating simulations involves multiple components. One component reflects students' performance and whether they met the objectives and demonstrated the skills and knowledge identified as important outcomes for that scenario. Another component is evaluation of the simulation itself and whether it met the objectives for which it was developed. As the simulation is running, it is possible to identify areas that are working and areas that are a challenge. The dynamic process of the simulation allows for some modification while it is running, but careful note taking during and after running the scenario as well as after the debriefing session with students will document changes necessary to enhance the effectiveness of the simulation. Finally, asking for student feedback both in the debriefing and anonymously in a written format will allow further revisions and improvement.

For student evaluation, computer-generated logs can be created by the automated setting of a high-fidelity HPS, with an option for the teacher to type comments while students are performing the scenario. In addition, video recording of the scenarios will provide concrete information about students' actions, knowledge, and skill. Evaluation can include the use of checklists, rating scales, or any other form for consistent scoring and grading among faculty members. Evaluation should be part of the template creation for each simulation.

SUMMARY

The use of clinical simulation in nursing education is increasing rapidly. There are a variety of methods, uses, and forms, but the major objective is to provide a safe, nonthreatening environment for students to learn clinical skills, critical thinking and decision making, and collaboration. Simulation is not new to the health care field, but with the advent of affordable equipment and user-friendly technology, more and more nursing education programs are exploring its use. The different levels of simulation, including low-, moderate-, and high-fidelity simulators, provide a variety of opportunities for learning. Beginner skills such as bed-making of occupied beds, sterile dressing changes, and catheterization can be practiced and learned on lower fidelity mannequins. High-fidelity human patient simulators provide interactive, realistic scenarios with changing physical attributes and actions in response to student interventions, and opportunities to practice real-time critical thinking and team work. The computer logs and recording of these scenarios provide concrete feedback for assessment and evaluation. Other types of simulation, including computer-assisted instruction, web technologies, and electronic medical records, also afford enhanced learning.

Nursing educators must weigh the advantages and challenges of incorporating simulation into their teaching. "Champion" faculty who are technologically competent and excited about the use of innovative teaching methodologies can motivate their colleagues to consider the possibilities of simulation-focused pedagogy. Further research on the efficacy and benefits of simulation are needed in all areas.

Implementation of simulation can progress from a simple to a complex level. Taking a visionary approach and identifying where simulation fits in the curriculum and the program, as well as setting up a process for assessment and evaluation, is ideal. Securing funding for faculty support in the form of consultants, conference attendance, and release time for course development will contribute to success.

The creation of simulation scenarios includes five characteristics: objectives, fidelity, complexity, cues, and debriefing/guided reflection. This chapter outlines these characteristics and gives examples of how to incorporate them in the creation of a scenario. Evaluation of simulation experiences includes multiple components such as student performance, actual running of the scenario, the success of the debriefing process, and student feedback on the simulation.

Suggestions for the planning of a simulation lab are provided. These include identifying uses of the lab, specialty environments, and a variety of resources.

Seeking funding for lab renovation, ensuring institutional support, and partnering with the community to provide services to staff members of health care organizations may be innovative ways to ensure development and sustainability of the simulation lab and its equipment. Finally, a commitment to faculty development and support for this pedagogical paradigm shift is of paramount importance.

Nurse educators encounter a variety of opportunities and challenges as they shift from didactic, content-focused teaching styles to a more dynamic, simulation-focused pedagogy for teaching. The learning curve for the development and running of scenarios may be high, but the outcomes in student learning and increased self-confidence as well as enhanced faculty–student interaction make the effort worthwhile. It is expected that clinical simulation will allow for increased ease of transition from student to employee roles, increased student comfort and competence with technology in the workplace, and improved patient safety.

REFERENCES

Appel, N., Campbell, S. H., Lynch, N., & Novotny, J. (2006, March). *Advisory board development and operation.* Paper presented at the AACN-NAP Conference, "Building Blocks for Success," Washington, DC.

Babenko-Mould, Y., Andrusyszyn, M., & Goldenberg, D. (2004). Effects of computer-based clinical conferencing on nursing students' self-efficacy. *Journal of Nursing Education, 43,* 149–155.

Berryman, J. F., Armstrong, G., & Zenoni, L. (2006, June). *Colorado's collaborative approach to develop a work, education and lifelong learning simulation center.* Paper presented at the 11th Biennial North American Learning Resource Centers Conference, "Nursing Education on the Move: Technology, Creativity, and Innovation," Philadelphia, PA.

Bond, W., Kostenbader, M., & McCarthy, J. (2001). Prehospital and hospital-based health care providers' experience with a human patient simulator. *Prehospital Emergency Care, 5,* 284–287.

CCNE. (2003). *Standards for accreditation of baccalaureate and graduate nursing programs.* Retrieved June 22, 2006, from http://www.aacn.nche.edu/Accreditation/NewStandards.htm

Chambers, K. (2006, June). *Simulation in nursing education: The basics.* Paper presented at the 4th Annual Laerdal® Northeast Simulation User's Group Meeting, Mashantucket, CT.

Clinton, J. (2006). Special delivery: Jefferson welcomes SimBaby. *Nursing Spectrum, Philadelphia Tri-State Edition, 15,* 16–17.

Collins, A., Edwards, R., & Graves, A. (2006). Dress rehearsal for critical care: Using a human patient simulator to augment clinical thinking. *Critical Care Nurse, 26,* S13.

Cooper, J., Barron, D., Blum, R., Davison, K., Feinstein, D., & Halasz, J. (2000). Video teleconferencing with realistic simulation for medical education. *Journal of Clinical Anesthesia, 12,* 256–261.

Donahue, B., & Thiede, K. (2006, June). *Integrating the electronic health record into high fidelity clinical simulations*. Paper presented at the 11th Biennial North American Learning Resource Centers Conference, "Nursing Education on the Move: Technology, Creativity, and Innovation," Philadelphia, PA.

Eichenwald, M. (2004). The ATHENS project: Advancing technology in health education at The College of St. Scholastica. *ADVANCE for Health Information Professionals: Issues in Education, 14*, 20.

Engum, S., & Jeffries, P. (2003). Intravenous catheter training system: Computer-based education vs. traditional learning methods. *The American Journal of Surgery, 186*, 67–74.

Freeman, K., Thompson, S., Allely, E., Sobel, A., Stansfield, S., & Pugh, W. (2001). A virtual reality patient simulation system for teaching emergency response skills to U.S. Navy medical providers. *Prehospital & Disaster Medicine, 16*, 3–8.

Fritzsche, D., Leonard, N., Boscia, M., & Anderson, P. (2004). Simulation debriefing procedures. *Developments in Business Simulation and Experiential Learning, 31*, 337–338.

Gaba, D. M., Howard, S., & Fish, K. (2001). Simulation-based training in anesthesia crisis management (ACRM): A decade of experience. *Simulation & Gaming, 32*, 175–193.

Goetz, M., & Nissen, H. (2005). Educational innovations. Building skills in pediatric nursing: Using a child care center as a learning laboratory. *Journal of Nursing Education, 44*, 277–279.

Goldenberg, D., Andrusyszyn, M., & Iwasiw, C. (2005). The effect of classroom simulation on nursing students' self-efficacy related to health teaching. *Journal of Nursing Education, 44*, 310–314.

Ham, K., & O'Rourke, E. (2004). Clinical strategies. Clinical preparation for beginning nursing students: An experiential learning activity. *Nurse Educator, 29*, 139–141.

Hamilton, R. (2005). Nurses' knowledge and skill retention following cardiopulmonary resuscitation training: A review of the literature. *Journal of Advanced Nursing, 51*, 288–297.

Haskvitz, L., & Koop, E. (2004). Educational innovations. Students struggling in clinical? A new role for the patient simulator. *Journal of Nursing Education, 43*, 181–184.

Henneman, E., & Cunningham, H. (2005). Using clinical simulation to teach patient safety in an acute/critical care nursing course. *Nurse Educator, 30*, 172–177.

Hertel, J., & Millis, B. (2002). *Using simulations to promote learning in higher education*. Sterling, VA: Stylus Publishing.

Hjelm-Karlsson, K., & Stenbeck, H. (1997). A simulation that teaches clinical decision making in nursing. In *Nursing informatics: The impact of nursing knowledge on health care informatics. Proceedings of NI'97, Sixth Triennial International Congress of IMIA-NI, Nursing Informatics of International Medical Informatics Association* (46th ed., pp. 492–495), Amsterdam, Netherlands: IOS Press.

Hravnak, M., Tuite, P., & Baldisseri, M. (2005). Expanding acute care nurse practitioner and clinical nurse specialist education: Invasive procedure training and human simulation in critical care. *AACN Clinical Issues: Advanced Practice in Acute & Critical Care, 16*, 89–104.

Jeffries, P. (2005). A framework for designing, implementing, and evaluating: Simulations used as teaching strategies in nursing. *Nursing Education Perspectives, 26*, 96–103.

Johnson-Russell, J., & Anderson, M. (2006, June). *Not just an afterthought: The art of debriefing/guided reflection.* Paper presented at the 11th Biennial North American Learning Resource Centers Conference, "Nursing Education on the Move: Technology, Creativity, and Innovation," Philadelphia, PA.

Jones, N. (2002). *The facilitation of interactive simulation.* Retrieved June 21, 2006, from http://www.patientsimulation.co.uk/4653/7006.html

Kappus, L., Leon, V., Lyons, A., Meehan, P., & Hamilton-Bruno, S. (2006). Simulation training: An innovative way to teach critical care nursing skills. *Critical Care Nurse*, 26(2), S15.

Kobayashi, L., Shapiro, M., Suner, S., & Williams, K. (2003). *Disaster medicine: The role of high fidelity medical simulation for mass casualty incident training.* Retrieved June 22, 2006, from http://www.findarticles.com/p/articles/mi_qa4100/is_200307/ai_n9268501/print

Kohn, L., Corrigan, J., & Donaldson, M. (2000). *To err is human: Building a safer health system.* Washington, D.C.: National Academy Press, Institute of Medicine.

Kurrek, M., & Fish, K. (1996). Anesthesia crisis resource management training: An intimidating concept, a rewarding experience. *Canadian Journal of Anesthesia*, 43(5, Part 1), 430–434.

Larew, C., Lessans, S., Spunt, D., Foster, D., & Covington, B. (2006). Innovations in clinical simulation: Application of Benner's theory in an interactive patient care simulation. *Nursing Education Perspectives*, 27, 16–21.

Long, R. (2005). Using simulation to teach resuscitation: An important patient safety tool. *Critical Care Nursing Clinics of North America*, 17(1), 1–8.

Madorin, S., & Iwasiw, C. (1999). The effects of computer-assisted instruction on the self-efficacy of baccalaureate nursing students. *Journal of Nursing Education*, 38, 282–285.

Marshall, R., Smith, J., Gorman, P., Krummel, T., Haluck, R., & Cooney, R. (2001). Use of a human patient simulator in the development of resident trauma management skills. *Journal of Trauma*, 51, 17–21.

McCartney, P. (2005). The new networking: Human patient simulators in maternal-child nursing. *MCN: The American Journal of Maternal Child Nursing*, 30, 215.

McCausland, L., Curran, C., & Cataldi, P. (2004). *Use of a human simulator for undergraduate nursing education.* Retrieved June 20, 2006, from http://www.bepress.com/ijnes/vol1/iss1/art23/

Morgan, P., Cleave-Hogg, D., McIlroy, J., & Devitt, J. (2002). Simulation technology: A comparison of experiential and visual learning for undergraduate medical students. *Anesthesiology*, 96, 10–16.

Morton, P. (1997). Academic education. Using a critical care simulation laboratory to teach students. *Critical Care Nurse*, 17, 66–69.

NCSBN. (2005). *NCSBN position paper: Clinical instruction in prelicensure nursing programs.* Retrieved June 20, 2006, from http://www.ncsbn.org/pdfs/Final_Clinical_Instr_Pre_Nsg_programs.pdf

Owens, L., & Walden, D. (2001). Peer instruction in the learning laboratory: A strategy to decrease student anxiety. *Journal of Nursing Education*, 40, 375–377.

Ravert, P. (2006, June). *Implementation of perinatal scenarios with use of high-fidelity patient simulator.* Paper presented at the 11th Biennial North American Learning Resource

Centers Conference, "Nursing Education on the Move: Technology, Creativity, and Innovation," Philadelphia, PA.

Rhodes, M., & Curran, C. (2005). Use of the human patient simulator to teach clinical judgment skills in a baccalaureate nursing program. *CIN: Computers, Informatics, Nursing, 23*, 256–264.

Russell, A., & Campbell, S. H. (2006, June 17). *Partnerships between nursing and technology.* Paper presented at the Partnerships in Progress, "Pathways to the Future in Nursing," Fairfield, CT.

Schumacher, L. (2004). *The impact of utilizing high-fidelity computer simulation on critical thinking abilities and learning outcomes in undergraduate nursing students.* Unpublished doctoral dissertation, Duquesne University, Pittsburgh, PA.

Seropian, M., Brown, K., Gavilanes, J., & Driggers, B. (2004a). An approach to simulation program development. *Journal of Nursing Education, 43*, 170–174.

Seropian, M., Brown, K., Gavilanes, J., & Driggers, B. (2004b). Simulation: Not just a manikin. *Journal of Nursing Education, 43*, 164–169.

Sheets, D. (2006, June). *Using a CIS format for case studies in classroom and simulated lab.* Paper presented at the 11th Biennial North American Learning Resource Centers Conference, "Nursing Education on the Move: Technology, Creativity, and Innovation," Philadelphia, PA.

Valentine, K. (2005). Electronic medical records promote caring and enhance professional vigilance. *International Journal for Human Caring, 9*, 121.

Weir, C., Hoffman, J., Nebeker, J., & Hurdle, J. (2005). Nurse's role in tracking adverse drug events: The impact of provider order entry. *Nursing Administration Quarterly, 29*, 39–44.

Yaeger, K., Halamek, L., Coyle, M., Murphy, A., Anderson, J., Boyle, K., et al. (2004). High-fidelity simulation-based training in neonatal nursing. *Advances in Neonatal Care, 4*, 326–331.

Chapter 10

Quality Clinical Education for Nursing Students at a Distance

Susan E. Stone and Mickey Gillmor-Kahn

Distance education has become a respected and effective method of providing undergraduate and graduate nursing education. In 2001, more than 51% of nursing education programs in the United States were using some type of distance education (Potempa, 2001). This percentage has expanded rapidly since then. Students choose distance education programs for a variety of reasons. These include issues related to distance from, and therefore limited access to, traditional university programs as well as the convenience of anytime, anyplace learning opportunities. Many distance-learning programs operate asynchronously, allowing students the ability to choose what time of the day or week they will participate. This flexibility makes distance-learning programs especially attractive to adult learners who may be working, raising families, or both while furthering their education. Many studies have shown that online learning is at least as effective as traditional classroom learning (American Association of Colleges of Nursing [AACN], 2000a).

But what about clinical education? The content in prelicensure and advanced practice nursing (APN) programs depends heavily on acquiring not only the didactic knowledge base but also a set of necessary clinical skills. Ultimately students must be able to demonstrate that they can apply the critical thinking process and function as safe, beginning-level practitioners in a clinical environment. This segment of their education cannot be completely taught or learned using computer technologies. This chapter provides some ideas and examples of how to design and implement an effective clinical education program that fits well with the distance education model, using the APN education programs at the Frontier School of Midwifery and Family Nursing (FSMFN) as an exemplar.

The effectiveness of prelicensure and APN education depends on the student being able to acquire clinical skills. When programs are offered at a distance, the availability of clinical sites and preceptors is required. It is best if the site is located in or near the student's own community. While nurse educators have been able to educate students who live almost anywhere using Internet technologies, often schools have only had affiliations with clinical sites located geographically close to their home base.

The FSMFN was faced with this dilemma in 1989, when we were transitioning our nurse-midwifery education program to a completely community-based model. The challenge was to build an effective program in which the student's own community could be used as a classroom. Since that time, FSMFN has graduated more than 1,000 nurse-midwives and nurse practitioners representing every state in the United States using a distance-education format.

A DESCRIPTION OF THE FRONTIER SCHOOL OF MIDWIFERY AND FAMILY NURSING

The FSMFN is a private, nonprofit, nonresidential, and community-based distance education graduate school. It offers a Master of Science in Nursing degree and post-master's certificates in specialty areas including nurse-midwife, family nurse practitioner, and women's health nurse practitioner. The mission of the school is to provide a high-quality education that prepares nurses to become competent, entrepreneurial, ethical, and compassionate nurse-midwives and nurse practitioners who will provide primary care for women and families. Our graduates serve those residing in all areas with a focus on rural and medically underserved populations. The program is designed to offer flexibility in graduate education for mature, self-directed adult learners who prefer independent study or who are unable to relocate to existing programs offering the nursing specialties provided in this program.

Our graduate program is based on the concept of community-based distance learning, a "university without walls." A core concept is that students learn best in their home environment. We strive not only to keep students in the communities that they plan to serve after graduation, but also to design learning activities that require students to examine the resources and needs of their communities. The community becomes a key learning environment.

All students begin their program of study by coming to the Hyden, Kentucky, campus to attend a 6-day orientation session we call "Frontier Bound." The orientation includes an introduction to all Level I courses by the faculty, meetings with their advisors, computer and library instruction, and, most important, establishing connections with each other as well as with the faculty and staff. With these connections students do not feel isolated when they return home. Students return to their communities where they complete Web-based courses for Level I, the foundational courses for practice, and Level II, the foundational courses for clinical management. Students interact with each other, faculty, staff, and alumni using the FSMFN Web portal system, named the "Banyan Tree," for course work, social support, and scholarly inquiry into practice issues. The students return to campus for Level III, a 2-week intensive skill training and verification of beginning clinical skills. Level IV focuses on clinical practice and the course work that is best suited for learning while in practice. Problem solving and developing independent decision-making skills are integral parts of the clinical practicum.

A challenge in the development of this program was to recruit excellent preceptors who were working in clinical sites that were geographically available to these distance learners. The first step was to identify potential preceptors in these communities. How could that be done? After much discussion, the conclusion was that the best person to identify clinical sites in the student's own community would be the student. Students were given basic guidelines regarding what was an acceptable preceptor site. The student had to locate a preceptor who was certified in the appropriate APN specialty. Amazingly enough, the system of students' identifying local preceptors has facilitated the establishment of more than 1,000 clinical sites across the United States. The plan worked and has continued to be effective for more than 15 years. Today the same process is used effectively for the nurse-midwifery, family nurse practitioner, and women's health nurse practitioner program options.

ESTABLISHING THE CLINICAL SITE

The process of securing a quality clinical site for each student is a lengthy endeavor. It includes a series of checks and balances designed to assure that students receive the education that they need and that the preceptor's needs for support, guidance in teaching, and rewards are met.

Identifying Potential Sites

First, the student identifies the preceptor. Preceptors are often identified through the health care organization where the student works, through local professional organization membership lists, through word of mouth, and sometimes even through the telephone book. Faculty members assist students in identifying appropriate sites by offering information about sites that have been used successfully in the past. We also provide guidance regarding site selection based on the student's interests or past experiences. For example, a midwifery student who only has experience in a high-risk obstetrical setting will be encouraged to seek out a low-risk setting such as a freestanding birthing center. In addition, school staff members provide lists of preceptor sites that hold contracts with the school in a specific geographic region. Students call preceptors to ask if they would be willing to consider precepting a student. If a practitioner is agreeable to exploring this arrangement, the student sends the preceptor's contact information to the school.

The school employs several Regional Clinical Coordinators (RCCs) who are the key to providing quality clinical learning opportunities for the student. The RCCs are faculty members who provide the essential link between the clinical site and the school. These are expert clinical faculty members whose main focus is the evaluation of clinical sites and mentoring of both students and preceptors through the clinical practica. Each RCC covers a specific geographic territory. Most RCCs are part-time faculty members who are expert clinicians in clinical practice in the region that they cover. Other faculty members do RCC work as a part of their full-time faculty workload. The fact that RCCs live in the region that they cover is an added benefit because they often know many of the providers and are aware of the regional issues that affect practice. The RCCs are paid on a per-event basis. They receive an hourly wage for travel and time at a clinical site plus all expenses. They also receive a fee for each student whose clinical activities they facilitate.

The school faculty has developed a packet of information describing the role of the clinical preceptor, clinical practicum requirements, Site Evaluation Report form, and required contract. The packet also contains a preceptor training course called "Act of Hope, Labor of Love: The Handbook for Precepting Frontier Students." This resource can be accessed at http://www.midwives.org/ActofHope/. The course is designed as a modular continuing education program and includes a DVD supplemental program. The training covers such topics as adult learning theory, learning styles, orienting the learner, teaching techniques, tips for successful precepting, evaluation, and dealing with difficulties in clinical teaching. In an attempt to meet preceptors' needs, the information is sent via mail and is also available via the FSMFN Web site.

On receiving notification from the student of a potential preceptor, a school staff member immediately sends a letter of introduction and a preceptor packet to the preceptor. The RCC follows up with a phone call to discuss the contents of the packet and the role of the preceptor. It is important to establish the best way to communicate with each preceptor. Some preceptors prefer telephone calls and some prefer e-mail. The preceptor is asked to complete a Site Evaluation Report. This form is designed to give the school information about the clinical site including location, number and type of clinicians, number and types of clients seen at that site, clinical learning opportunities available for the student, and the type of site (hospital clinic, rural health clinic, freestanding birth center, and others).

Preclinical Site Visit

The next step is a preclinical site visit done by the RCC. The RCC goes to the clinical site to evaluate the practice for its educational potential in preparing nurse-midwifery or nurse practitioner students and to orient the preceptor to the teaching role. The site visit is held on a typical clinical day providing the opportunity for the RCC to see the practice in action.

The RCC completes the following activities at a preclinical site visit:

- A tour of the physical facilities including the hospital or birth center
- A review of the practice guidelines to confirm that they are current and appropriate;
- A review of a sample of client records completed by the preceptor
- A review, with the preceptors, of all FSMFN policies and materials regarding students and the clinical experience
- An opportunity for the preceptors to ask any questions they may have

Contractual Arrangements With Clinical Sites

The contract between the school and the clinical site specifies the responsibilities of each participant. The school has a standard contract that is sent with the information packet. In many cases the contract is signed and sent back without question. In some cases, the site will send back its own contract and request that school officials sign it. In that case, the school officials and lawyers review the proposed contract to make sure it meets the school's requirements. This can be a lengthy process. If the student will be participating in clinical experiences in both a clinic and a hospital that are separate entities, then two separate contracts may be required.

It is important that the contract address, at minimum, the following issues: First, the student will be under the guidance of the preceptor. It should be clear in the contract that the preceptor is the faculty member and there will not be another faculty member from the school on-site to instruct and evaluate the student. Second, both the school and the clinical site must carry a program of insurance. The FSMFN requires sites to have at least the same amount of coverage as the FSMFN. Certificates of insurance are exchanged by the school and the clinical site as a part of the contractual agreement.

Third, a bilateral indemnity clause should be included in the contract such as the following:

> SCHOOL will defend, indemnify, and hold the Agency harmless from any and all losses, claims, liabilities, damages, costs, and expenses (including reasonable attorney's fees) to the extent caused solely by the negligence of SCHOOL, its agents, employees, or students in connection with this Agreement or by any breach or default in the performance of the obligations of SCHOOL hereunder.
>
> CLINICAL SITE will defend, indemnify, and hold SCHOOL harmless from any and all losses, claims, liabilities, damages, costs, and expenses (including reasonable attorney's fees) to the extent caused solely by the negligence of the Agency, its agents, employees, or students in connection with this Agreement or by any breach or default in the performance of the obligations of the Agency hereunder.

Fourth, the contract should include language specifying that the student and RCC have been trained in Health Insurance Portability and Accountability Act of 1996 (HIPAA) rules and regulations and will abide by the same. Finally, there should be language stating that the clinical site and its staff retain full responsibility for the care of its patients. For example: "Nothing in this Agreement shall be construed to shift the ultimate responsibility for patient care from the Agency, its physicians, and its other health care professionals."

The school has a quality assurance coordinator (QAC) who attends to all the clinical contracts and maintains the credentials of preceptors and all other required quality checks. In some cases, the QAC must consult with the School's legal counsel regarding certain contract issues. These issues can be complex due to the fact that we are dealing with students from all 50 states, and regulations are often different from state to state. The FSMFN students are not allowed to provide care at a clinical site until the contract is in place. They may visit the site to observe but are instructed that they may not participate in clinical care until the contract is signed.

PRECEPTORS

The Preceptor Interview

Preceptors should have a face-to-face interview with every student prior to agreeing to the precepting arrangement. Many misunderstandings, including misperceptions about the skills, abilities, and past experience of a particular student, can be avoided with good preparation. Prior to meeting with the preceptor, the student completes a clinical skills checklist and submits it along with a current curriculum vitae to the preceptor. The clinical skills checklist details the clinical skills that will be required during the experience. Students identify whether they have no experience, some experience, or a lot of experience with each particular skill. In the adult learning model, students bring a wide variety of skills to the learning experience. This list helps the preceptor to discern a particular student's skill level in different areas.

The FSMFN student then makes an appointment to meet with the preceptor. The overall purpose of the meeting is for the preceptor to interview the student, explain the logistics of the clinical site, and determine whether there is a good match between the student and the preceptor. The preceptor is encouraged to ask many questions of the student and is given a form to guide the interview.

Sample questions may include:

Why do you want to be a CNM/FNP/Women's Health Care Nurse Practitioner (WHCNP)?

What advanced practice settings have you been exposed to in the past and in what capacity?

How do you respond when someone critiques your performance?

Tell me why we should agree to precept you.

Do you anticipate any constraints on your time when you are in the clinical setting?

The preceptor also informs the student of the responsibilities at this site, including expectations for arrival, dress, and schedule. If there seems to be a good match at the end of the interview, the preceptor completes the preceptor interview form and submits it to the school with a signed agreement stating that the preceptor has agreed to precept this student.

Credentialing of Preceptors

Once the preceptor agrees to precept the student, the credentialing process begins. Requirements of the process are defined by the school's accrediting agencies. In the case of FSMFN, these include the American College of Nurse-Midwives Division of Accreditation, the National League for Nursing Accrediting Commission, and the Southern Association of Colleges and Schools. Credentialing is an important process because students must be assured that they are receiving instruction from qualified faculty. The preceptors are appointed as clinical faculty of the school. They must submit their original transcripts, their curricula vitae, and copies of their professional nursing licenses to the school.

Most preceptors are not happy about this paperwork, so FSMFN strives to make it as easy as possible. For example, the QAC can now check a preceptor's current license in most states through an online search. If the preceptor completes the release form for the original transcript and returns it to the school, the QAC completes the transcript request to the preceptor's school of graduation and FSMFN pays the transcript fees. Clinical faculty members must also complete teaching preparation. They can do this by completing the modules included in the FSMFN Preceptor Packet or by using other available online resources developed by other schools and professional organizations (Raisler, O'Grady, & Lori, 2003). They may also attend teacher training offered at regional or national conferences.

Preceptor Honoraria

Providing monetary compensation to clinical preceptors has been debated and has even become a contentious issue because some programs are prohibited from doing so by the organizational rules of their parent university (Raisler, O'Grady, et al., 2003). When sending students out to distance sites where the preceptor will have primary responsibility for the student's clinical education, some form of preceptor compensation should be considered. If a school cannot offer monetary compensation, other rewards should be considered such as free continuing education contact hours or access to online library resources. Often the preceptors are in remote sites and greatly appreciate such services. Acknowledgement of the critical role of preceptors in teaching students can help preceptors feel valued and appreciated.

STUDENT CLINICAL LEARNING ACTIVITIES

Activities Prior to Beginning Clinical Practice

All of the preparatory work for clinical learning activities is accomplished during the 12 to 18 months when FSMFN students are completing their Level I, II, and III courses. Students return to campus for the 2-week Level III session. Level III is held five times each year so that as students complete Level II at their own pace, they can register to attend Level III.

Level III focuses on refining and using the knowledge that students have acquired during their online studies. Students practice physical exam skills, microscope skills, and suturing skills. They also do role-plays and interactive case studies in a classroom with FSMFN faculty. They use simulators to practice all types of physical exams skills such as Leopold maneuvers, heart and lung exam, breast exam, and prostate exam. The pregnant Noelle® Maternal and Neonatal Birthing Simulator (Laerdal/Medical) allows midwifery students to practice the hand skills necessary to assist a woman in childbirth.

Students also have observational activities with faculty members from the faculty practice in the Frontier Nursing Service rural health clinics. They visit the home of Mary Breckinridge and learn more about the history of the Frontier Nursing Service and its meaning to the development of advanced practice nursing in the United States. Students' health records are checked to assure that they have all the required immunizations and the like prior to starting clinical learning activities. Students review the clinical contract with the QAC so that they clearly know what the site requirements are. They also participate in sessions on HIPAA and Occupational Safety and Health Administration (OSHA) regulations.

The last Level III session that students attend prior to returning home and starting their clinical learning activities is "Transition to Clinical Practice." In this class they learn about expectations in the clinical setting, clinical evaluation tools, and the requirements regarding completing daily, weekly, and monthly evaluation tools. At the end of Level III, students are ready to return to their communities and begin Level IV and clinical learning activities.

A preclinical meeting between the student and the preceptor should occur before the student starts any clinical activity. A substantial amount of time may have elapsed between the preceptor interview and the student having completed Level III. Both student and preceptor need to be brought up-to-date. During this meeting, the student and preceptor should discuss the following items:

- The student's background, progress through the program, and any special areas identified as needing the attention of the preceptor.

- A plan for orientation to each clinical setting and any documentation and credentialing that the site requires, such as copies of the nursing license, proof of immunity to rubella or other diseases, facility personnel identification badge, keys, and so on. Directions to each site and parking information also are helpful.

- The Practice Guidelines for the type of practice in which the student will participate. It is desirable for the student to make or purchase a copy to review and carry. If there are no specific written guidelines, the protocol or resources that the preceptor uses should be identified for the student.

- Appropriate professional attire for the settings.

- How to communicate with the preceptor if ill or unable to attend a clinical learning activity for another urgent reason.

- Introduction to or description of other providers in the practice, and any relevant issues concerning their needs and availability.

- Any expectations and opportunities for attending staff meetings, case reviews, grand rounds, and so forth.

- Any special considerations in dealing with clients or with hospital, office, or clinic personnel.

Schedule and Assignments

Students start the clinical practicum with many different levels of expertise. Some feel confident and some are anxious. We have found that the following recommendations help students and preceptors begin clinical teaching and learning activities on solid ground.

- Students begin in the setting with a single preceptor. Although there may be several preceptors at a site, it is best if the student spends a minimum of 2 weeks with one preceptor prior to spending time with another in that site.
- Some observation time should be built into the first few days of clinical learning activities. Even though some students may be eager to jump in and get started, an initial period of observation is strongly recommended. Observing helps the student to understand the environment and role expectations of the particular setting.
- Preceptors should bring a clinical schedule to the first meeting, show it to the student, and plan a schedule for the first 3 to 4 weeks. Depending on the structure of the educational program, students may still have course work to complete, and therefore, may need to limit the amount of time spent in the clinical setting. Others will have completed their course work and will be able to make a full-time commitment to clinical practice.
- The preceptor should review the student's expectations for the clinical placement including when he or she plans to finish and what he or she hopes to accomplish at the site. In addition, the requirements of the educational program should be reviewed.

Length of Clinical Placement

The length of the clinical placement will be defined by the educational program. Most prelicensure and APN programs will have a required number of hours that students must spend in clinical practice. Many also will have a required number of specific clinical activities that the student must complete.

For example, at FSMFN all students must complete 675 hours of clinical practice. The nurse-midwifery students must also complete the following activities:

- 10 preconception care visits,

- 30 new antepartum visits,

- 140 return antepartum visits,

- 40 labors managed,

- 40 births (which may include 4 observations),

- 40 newborn assessments,

- 20 breast-feeding support visits,

- 40 postpartum visits (2 hours to 14 days postpartum),

- 30 postpartum visits (2 to 8 weeks postpartum),

- 40 common health problems,

- 30 family planning visits,

- 25 non-postpartum gynecologic visits,

- 25 perimenopausal/postmenopausal visits.

Some of these categories overlap, and a single visit may therefore count in more than one category.

The Family Nurse Practitioner students must complete the following activities:

- 10 new antepartum visits,

- 30 returning antepartum visits,

- 50 speculum/bimanual exam,

- 10 newborn exams,

- 30 infant/toddler exams,

- 30 school-age exams,

- 10 adolescent exams,

- 300 client visits for episodic or wellness care,

- 150 client visits for chronic illness care.

Not all clinical sites will be able to provide the required number of clinical learning activities in all areas. Some students need to work with more than one preceptor to complete these required activities. An interview, orientation, and observation period will be appropriate at the beginning of work at each new clinical site.

Engaging the Student Academically While in the Clinical Area

The FSMFN students must be able to complete the required Level IV course work and complete their clinical practicum at the same time. This dual objective can be very challenging. It is imperative that preceptors have a good understanding of what is required of the student. Written materials, both as paper documents and online, provided to the preceptor can help to accomplish this goal. We have found that preceptors like the paper version initially so that they can sit down and read through it. Having the document online provides ready access to the information if the preceptor would like to refer to it at some future point when the paper copy is not at hand.

In addition to the written material, it is helpful for the school faculty to explain to the preceptor exactly what is expected of the student when starting clinical practice. At Frontier, RCCs either talk to or e-mail preceptors (some communicate very well with e-mail and others need to hear a voice on the telephone) every 2 weeks about the student's progress and the expectations of the next 2 weeks. At the beginning of the clinical practicum, students are expected to do less clinical practice and more course work. For example, they may attend the clinical site 2 or 3 days per week. Later when the course work is completed, they will do a full schedule of clinical care.

Courses that students complete at the same time that they have clinical practice are developed with specific goals that include relating the clinical experience with the course work and facilitating student interactions. Strategies that encourage student-to-student interactions and faculty–student interactions are critical to learning success (Mueller & Billings, 2005). In a distance-learning environment, developing strategies to achieve these interactions takes careful planning. Faculty members at FSMFN have developed assignments that require students not only to use their experiences in clinical practice to complete learning activities, but also to share these experiences with their classmates. For example, one assignment that midwifery students complete is called "Listen to Women." They must interview a woman about her experience of pregnancy and then post the interview in the class forum. Other students respond with thoughtful questions and comments about the interview. Students receive credit for both their original posting and their responses to other students' postings.

Another assignment requires students to present in the course online forum an interesting case that they have seen in their clinical experience. Each student chooses a client who experienced a complication or variation of normal. Variations can include medical or psychosocial issues. The student briefly presents the relevant background information on the client: basic identifying information (using initials or a pseudonym to protect the client's identity) and pertinent historical information. The student describes the complication or variation of normal, its presentation, and any related risk factors present. The student then opens the case for discussion by indicating questions for the respondents to consider, for example, Do you agree with the assessment made? Do you agree that this situation requires intervention?

All students and faculty are welcome to comment and participate in discussion. Each student actively enrolled in this course is required to post a thoughtful response to at least one case presentation. The presenter is then required to discuss the responses, the actual management, the outcome, and what he or she learned from this situation. Students receive credit for both their presentation and their responses to others' presentations.

These activities provide a variety of benefits. They supplement student learning. They help students at a distance maintain contact with the learning community. They provide an outlet for discussion and examination of complex clinical situations with their faculty and fellow students. The faculty strives to maintain a supportive environment in course forums so that students feel safe in openly discussing their experiences and their questions about the experience.

Choosing the Precepting Style

Preceptor and student need to communicate well regarding competence, confidence, and commitment so that an appropriate precepting style can be selected. Blanchard's styles of leadership and developmental levels can be helpful in thinking about choices of precepting styles. Blanchard, Zigarmi, and Zigarmi, (1985) described a method of adapting one's leadership style to the needs of those being led. As people learn new skills they proceed through four developmental levels. The developmental level is determined by one's competence (skills and knowledge) and commitment (confidence and enthusiasm). The levels are

- D1, enthusiastic and ready to learn,

- D2, some disillusionment and decreased commitment as one learns that the task is more difficult than expected,

- D3, learning continues with increased knowledge and skills, and commitment fluctuates from excitement to insecurity,

- D4, high level of competence, motivation, and commitment.

Leaders should adapt their style of leadership to match the developmental level. Leadership styles include S1, Directing; S2, Coaching; S3, Supporting; and S4, Delegating (Blanchard, et al., 1985). At FSMFN, we have found that Blanchard's model works well when precepting students.

Students move through the developmental levels from enthusiastic beginner with little knowledge but high motivation, to intermediate levels of competence and often less motivation, to finally achieving a level of competence in which ideally both skills and motivation are high. Precepting styles should adjust to the needs of the student at each level of competence and commitment. Early on students need specific direction, time to observe, and careful coaching. As students progress, the preceptor gives less direction and allows them more independence while still providing support and encouragement. For specific new skill acquisition, the preceptor reverts to a more directive or coaching style as the situation demands.

Cultural and learning style differences may also need to be taken into consideration. Some students will be impatient with a request to observe, wanting to jump in right away and perform tasks. Others will be reluctant to step in until they have observed the preceptor's methods and interactions several times. Some students will need to be encouraged to apply their knowledge; others may need direction to find the learning available while observing a skilled practitioner.

STUDENT EVALUATION

Evaluating students while in clinical practice is an ongoing challenge for preceptors and school faculty members. Goals of evaluation (Table 10.1) include identification of student strengths and problem areas as well as documentation of student progress. In addition, evaluation of student competence and commitment can assist the preceptor in selecting an appropriate precepting style.

Evaluation in a distance setting has its own challenges. School faculty members must develop a working relationship with clinical preceptors who are at a distance. Contact between the faculty and the preceptor during the student's clinical activities experience needs to be timely and consistent. Preceptors need to know how to reach the designated school faculty member for concerns and support. At the same time, teaching and student evaluation can be time-consuming, and the school needs to avoid imposing unnecessary additional reporting burdens on

TABLE 10.1   Goals of Clinical Evaluation

Identification of student strengths
Identification of areas in which the student needs more experience and support
Identification of serious deficiencies
Documentation of the strengths and areas for improvement as they are identified
Documentation of the resolution of problem areas
Identification of the level of student competence
Identification of the level of student confidence and commitment
Documentation of student clinical learning activities and hours

the preceptor. When working at a distance, e-mail communication can be helpful to busy preceptors and faculty alike, as long as all is going well. When problems arise there is no substitute for direct communication by phone, and if necessary, in person.

Tools for Student Evaluation

Various tools have been developed by schools to assist in the evaluation process. The FSMFN believes that student self-evaluation is essential and requires written evaluation and reflection on clinical experiences on a daily basis. This daily exercise provides a venue for mature self-evaluation and plans for improvement. The student's self-evaluation is shared with the preceptor who may comment or add suggestions and signs the daily form. Involvement of the preceptor in daily written assessments provides oversight and documentation. The form used by FSMFN students to document this daily evaluation is called the Daily Developmental Assessment Tool (DDAT). While self-identification of areas needing improvement can be stressful for students, we believe that this self-critique is the basis for a mature practitioner's growth and should be fostered by the educational program.

The FSMFN also requires a Monthly Developmental Assessment Tool (MDAT). This tool allows the student and preceptor to review and document the student's progress in a more specific format. The MDATs describe domains of learning with specific behaviors to be accomplished in each domain. Because four stages are delineated, the student and preceptor are able to see and document student progress toward independence. Both the DDAT and the MDAT forms may be viewed at the FSMFN Web site (http://www.midwives.org/actofhope/ 7AppendD.shtm). All forms are sent to the RCC monthly who reviews them to assess overall progress. In addition, the RCC talks with the student by phone at least every other week during the clinical practicum.

Clinical Site Visit

An important element of the evaluation of student performance occurs at a clinical site visit. At the FSMFN, all students routinely receive an on-site, in-person visit from their RCC during their clinical practicum. Ideally this visit is scheduled midway through the clinical period. It provides an opportunity for the RCC to assess and support the student and the preceptor. It also prevents the student from feeling that the visit is a "final exam" and provides time for remediation if necessary. The purposes of the clinical site visit are to

- provide supplemental and formative evaluation of the student's clinical progress, including documentation in client records;

- assess the teaching relationship between student and preceptor;

- foster on-going development of preceptors as instructors;

- provide support and information to the FSMFN student and clinical faculty.

The RCC makes the appointment with the practice director or the student's primary preceptor, as appropriate, at some time after the student has been in the clinical practicum. Scheduling site visits is an important issue. The site visit must be scheduled at a time that is mutually agreeable to the student, the preceptor, and the RCC. The RCCs very often travel long distances to attend a site visit. It is not unusual for air travel to be required. Preceptors need to be aware of this travel component when the visit is being arranged so that they commit completely to that date, knowing it will not be an easy issue to reschedule.

Written confirmation of the details and plans for the site visit, its date, time, location, and the needed materials, should be sent to both preceptor and student at least 1 month ahead of time. Clients should be informed that a site visit is planned and given the opportunity to decline participation.

Observation of Student During the Site Visit.   The RCC observes while the student and preceptor see clients in the clinical site. The role of the RCC is one of observer. It is important to be clear that the preceptor is responsible for the care given and for the teaching. The RCC as site visitor may offer advice and praise as appropriate. Comments or suggestions about the care given can be shared with the student, preferably after the day is over or at a lunch break.

Students are typically quite nervous during a site visit and allowance needs to be made for that nervousness. After a few client encounters with the RCC observing, the student usually begins to relax. A few well-chosen words of praise early on can help.

Ideally the clinical site schedule should include a variety of patient types. For nurse-midwifery students this variety would include an initial pregnancy exam, return prenatal visits at various gestations, postpartum/family planning visits, well woman, and newborn checks, if applicable. For FNP students, health mainte-nance visits, acute visits, and chronic visits including follow-up visits with clients of a variety of ages and both genders would provide variety.

Meeting With Student and Preceptor During the Site Visit. The RCC also plans time to meet separately with the preceptor and with the student; to tour the facilities in-cluding the hospital or birth center, if applicable; and to review the nurse-midwifery practice or nurse practitioner guidelines/protocols and student charting from all settings. Scheduled time alone with the RCC gives the preceptor an opportunity to ask questions, discuss student progress, present any issues or concerns, and re-ceive information about teaching and learning styles, precepting styles, develop-mental stages, and expectations of the school for clinical faculty.

The RCC meets separately with the student to give feedback regarding chart-ing, clinical, and communication skills. Plans for the remainder of the student's clinical learning activities are developed with the student and the preceptor.

Case Presentation During the Site Visit. The site visit also provides an opportunity for the student to do a formal case presentation for the RCC. Students need to be advised of this requirement ahead of time and provided with guidelines so they can prepare. Nurse-midwifery students are asked to present an intrapartum case. Nurse practitioner students present an interesting case from their clinical experi-ence. The case should include some problematic aspect, which could be psycho-social or physical, but should focus on the issues manageable by the nurse-midwife or nurse practitioner, not simply referral to medical management.

Evaluation of Student Charting During the Site Visit. Evaluation of student chart-ing occurs during the clinical site visit by the FSMFN RCC. The RCC also reviews charting soon after the student begins clinical practice and until the preceptor and the school faculty member agree that the student is charting appropriately. The FSMFN requires students to write SOAP (subjective data, objective data, as-sessment, plan) notes on each client encounter at the time of the encounter. The preceptor reviews the SOAP note and cosigns. The note is then placed either in the chart or in a student notebook for review by the RCC at the time of the site visit.

Each month the student sends the RCC copies of two SOAP notes from each type of clinical encounter (names removed). Students are instructed to send actual SOAP notes written in the clinical setting, not rewritten or typed notes. Al-though the RCC is not present daily with students in the clinical situation, eval-uation of SOAP charting allows the RCC, as well as the preceptor, to see students' thought processes and improve their charting skills while helping them to mature as practitioners.

When reviewing SOAP charting off-site, the RCC is able to assess whether students are gathering appropriate data, how they interpret the data, and whether the plans are appropriate to the students assessment. Despite instruction and practice in SOAP charting during the academic portions of the program, many students still struggle with differentiating data collection (subjective and objective) from interpretation (assessment) and both of these from the plan of care for the client. Frequently the SOAP note will have a plan but no data, suggesting that a plan is needed, or the note may show data and even an assessment of a problem, but no plan. Through pointed questions and suggestions, the RCC can help students see the deficiencies in their charting and why complete documentation is important.

Because mature practitioners often do not provide full SOAP charting, the student may likewise not be producing complete SOAP notes. Often students model their charting on what the preceptor does, not recognizing that for educational purposes the school requires more documentation. Increasingly funding sources are also requiring more documentation than has been prevalent in the past. Thorough SOAP notes can also provide the documentation needed for billing purposes. In sites where charting is done by checklists or a computerized database, requiring students to do some handwritten SOAP notes still allows the preceptor and RCC to assess the student's internal processes of data collection, assessment, and planning.

Site Visit Report

Site visit reporting is important to the educational goals and evaluation. The site visit report should be filed promptly and shared with appropriate faculty members and administrative personnel, as well as filed with the student's records at the school. If any significant site or student problems are identified, the school faculty member needs to consult promptly with the program director, the student's advisor, or others as designated by the school.

DIAGNOSIS AND REMEDIATION OF LEARNING DIFFICULTIES DURING CLINICAL PRACTICE

The Problem ID Process

Students in distance education have learning issues similar to those of students in on-site educational programs. Recognizing them and finding ways to help the student overcome them at a distance present special challenges. The FSMFN has developed a tool for this purpose, which has proven helpful. When a preceptor, student, or the RCC recognizes a problem, the FSMFN Problem ID Sheet is used. This form may be accessed at the FSMFN Web site (http://www.midwives.org/actofhope/7AppendD.shtm).

The student and preceptor each fill out a Problem ID Sheet separately, then meet to discuss their responses. Their joint Problem ID Sheet is then forwarded to the RCC. When both student and preceptor can agree on the problem, its domain, and possible solutions, there may be no need for further intervention. Frequently, simply naming the problem and thinking about solutions together is enough to accomplish the goal.

For example, a student told the RCC that she felt that the preceptors were "breathing down her neck," did not allow her to do anything on her own, were treating her "like a baby," and were hypercritical of her care. The preceptors believed that the student did not understand her role, was arrogant, did procedures without supervision, and resented their teaching. They were on the verge of telling the student that she could not work with their clients any longer.

The RCC recommended that they each do a Problem ID Sheet and then meet to discuss the problems. Both student and preceptors agreed that there was a communication problem regarding the student's independence or dependence; that the student was critical about her own performance; and that instead of allowing herself time to learn, she expected herself to be an accomplished practitioner. Through the Problem ID process, the student came to recognize that her role as a student was different from her role as a staff nurse, and that instruction and evaluation were part of the process rather than a criticism of her skills. The student also acknowledged the preceptors' primary role with the clients and their need to protect both the clients and their practice.

For their part, the preceptors recognized that they were inconsistent in their instructions and expectations of the student. Their previous student had just graduated and was highly accomplished. They initially and unconsciously expected the current student to have the same skills as a previous student did just before graduation and were frustrated with the need to give such close and specific direction. Recognizing that the student needed more supervision than the previous one, they then overcompensated and did not allow the student any decision making at all.

Having identified these issues, student and preceptors, with the RCC's guidance, were then able to set a plan in place in which the student agreed not to do anything without specific approval of the preceptors, and the preceptors agreed to allow her to propose more of the plan of care with each client. Discussion with the RCC helped the student recognize that she was not an independent practitioner at that point in her education and that she could allow herself the time to learn without expecting perfection.

Expert-to-novice conflicts are common for experienced nurses returning to graduate school in which they are once again beginners (Forbes, 2004). At the same

TABLE 10.2   Learning Plan

1. Identify the problem.
2. Identify the resources necessary to solve the problem.
3. Set measurable goals.
4. Evaluate goals at least weekly.

Note: Generated by the student with faculty assistance.

time the preceptors learned through discussions with the student and the RCC that this student needed clear guidelines about expectations to form her own plan for discussion with the preceptors, they also became aware that her rapid-fire speech pattern was a cultural difference that did not necessarily mean that she was hostile.

The student developed a learning plan describing her current view of the problem (Table 10.2), the plan for remediation, and a date for another discussion to review the situation. Frequent communication with the RCC helped both student and preceptors through this transition period. In the end, communication improved as the result of this intervention, the student was clear about her boundaries in this role, the preceptors recognized the student's current developmental stage, and the student was able to remain in the site to complete her clinical learning activities.

Unresolved Problems: Problem Site Visits and Performance Plans

When the student and preceptors cannot agree on the problem, when one or the other does not believe there is a problem, or when the Problem ID and Learning Plan process do not result in an improvement in the situation, then further intervention from the school is necessary.

An emergency site visit allows the RCC to assess the situation in person, to facilitate a discussion between preceptor and student, and, if the problem is in motor skills or knowledge base domains, to observe the student's skills and interactions. In these circumstances the site visitor will not have the luxury of many weeks of advance planning. Flexibility in scheduling can be crucial, putting pressure on the school to accommodate this requirement. For this type of site visit, the goal is a clear discussion of the student's and the preceptor's views of the situation. The RCC acts as a facilitator for the discussion, helping the preceptor and student communicate the issues, and if possible, develop a plan for remediation.

After discussions with the preceptors and the student, the RCC and the Department Chair develop a Performance Plan for the student (Table 10.3). It

TABLE 10.3   Performance Plan

1. Identifies the problem.
2. Identifies specific behaviors that are expected from the student.
3. Sets dates for accomplishment of each behavior.
4. Sets evaluation dates.

Note: Developed by the faculty member for the student.

delineates expected behaviors in specific terms, specifies deadlines for accomplishment of the goals, and sets a date for review. The content of the Performance Plan should be as specific as possible and dates for review should be adhered to.

When preceptors and students disagree, at times it can seem impossible to determine the reality of the situation. Sometimes it becomes apparent that the best solution will be to transfer the student to a different site to allow other preceptors to perform an assessment. Occasionally the student will need to relocate to attend this new clinical site. This move is difficult for both the student and new preceptor, but can mean the difference between graduation and withdrawal of a student. Preceptors who are willing to take on students with problems for assessment and disposition should be treasured.

Rarely, problems cannot be resolved and the student simply needs to withdraw from the program. When that happens, clear and specific documentation of the student's problems becomes critical to help the student understand the problem and to avoid litigation. The careful use of evaluation tools throughout all students' clinical experience can avoid major problems in these difficult situations.

CLOSING THE LOOP ON CLINICAL EVALUATION

The clinical learning activities must be evaluated at each step of the program. This starts with the preclinical site visit to evaluate the learning environment at the clinical site. Can the site meet the needs of the student? Evaluation continues as the student completes daily evaluations that are reviewed by the preceptor. The monthly evaluation meeting between the student and the preceptor provides a checkpoint at which both the student and preceptor can evaluate the student's overall progress and set new goals for the coming month. Having the student send these evaluations to the RCC monthly allows the RCC to review the student's progress and the documentation. Having the students track their clinical hours and the number of learning activities completed assures that they have the necessary volume of clinical encounters. The clinical site visit allows the RCC to evaluate the progress of the student and the interactions of student and preceptor.

Students are ready to end the clinical practicum when they have completed all of the required clinical hours and learning activities and are functioning at Stage Four in all objectives listed on the monthly evaluation tool. At FSMFN, preceptors are asked to sign a Declaration of Safety form, which states that the student is functioning as a safe, beginning level practitioner. Preceptors are sent an evaluation tool designed to assess their satisfaction with the clinical site visit and their overall experience working with the school faculty. Students are asked to evaluate their preceptors, the learning activities at the clinical site, and the RCC. All of these evaluations assist the school in assessing and improving the effectiveness of clinical education.

GOALS FOR THE FUTURE

The FSMFN is currently working on the planning and implementation of a project for students to use a personal data assistant (PDA) during their clinical education. The plan is to issue a PDA to each student at the start of clinical learning activities. The PDAs will be loaded with software designed to provide access to clinical reference material and to track clinical encounters. Students will use the PDAs to access reference material while completing their clinical practica. In addition, students will enter the types of clients seen, the types of procedures completed, and the number of hours spent in the clinical setting each day. Students will dock the PDA at least weekly to send the information to the school. Faculty will then have access to the information. This will allow RCCs and Department Chairs to easily track the progress of each student in the clinical environment.

SUMMARY

Planning, supervising, and evaluating the clinical learning activities for distance learners provides challenges for administration, faculty, clinical preceptors, and students. Effective planning and attention to the importance of communication can overcome many of the challenges inherent in distance education and can sometimes offer students and preceptors support they might not find in an on-site experience. This chapter describes the use of a distance education format at one community-based graduate program in nursing, the Frontier School of Midwifery and Family Nursing (FSMFN).

The process of clinical teaching in a distance education program begins with identification of an appropriate preceptor and practice site for the student. The creation of a regional clinical coordinator position at the FSMFN has facilitated effective evaluation of potential clinical sites and orientation of preceptors and students to their respective roles.

Effective planning for clinical teaching and learning at a distance includes contractual arrangements with each clinical site that addresses relevant legal and quality assurance issues. Preparation and credentialing of preceptors and some form of compensation for their service are important considerations. Student learning activities may start with simulations and observation of faculty practice, and progress to clinical practice with their preceptors. Suggestions were made for optimum length and scheduling of clinical activities and for engaging students academically to facilitate acquisition of desired competencies. Appropriate written assignments and online clinical discussions and conferences enhance the clinical learning in distance education programs. A model of leadership behavior was suggested for use in choosing appropriate precepting styles for various levels of learners.

Clinical evaluation of students presents a challenge to most preceptors, especially in a distance education program. Suggestions were made for timely and consistent communication among faculty member, preceptor, and student to facilitate effective feedback about student performance. Clinical evaluation methods for various uses were described, including self-evaluation, documentation of student progress toward independence, on-site observation of student performance, and review of students' charting. Processes for identification and remediation of learning difficulties during clinical practice and for resolving conflicts between student and preceptor were presented.

REFERENCES

American Association of Colleges of Nursing. (2000a). *Distance learning is changing and challenging nursing education*. Retrieved November 2, 2005, from www.aacn.nche.edu/Publications/positions/issues/jan2000.htm

American Association of Colleges of Nursing. (2000b). *AACN white paper: Distance technology in nursing education*. Retrieved November 2, 2005, from www.aacn.nche.edu/Publications/positions/whitepaper.htm

Blanchard, K., Zigarmi, P., & Zigarmi, D. (1985). *Leadership and the one-minute manager: Increasing effectiveness through situational leadership*. New York: William Morrow and Company.

Forbes, V. J. (2004). From expert to novice: The unnerving transition from experienced RN to neophyte APN. *Journal of Holistic Nursing, 22*, 180–185.

Mueller, C., & Billings, D. (2005). Supporting learner success. In J. Novotny & R. Davis (Eds.), *Distance education in nursing* (2nd ed., pp. 47–68). New York: Springer Publishing.

Potempa, K. (2001). Where winds the road of distance education in nursing? *Journal of Nursing Education, 40*, 291–292.

Raisler, J., O'Grady, M., & Lori, J. (2003). Clinical teaching and learning in midwifery and women's health. *Journal of Midwifery and Women's Health, 48*, 398–406.

Chapter 11

Case Method, Case Study, and Grand Rounds

Clinical practice provides opportunities for students to gain the knowledge and skills needed to care for patients; develop values important in professional practice; and develop cognitive skills for processing and analyzing data, deciding on problems and interventions, and evaluating their effectiveness. Ability to apply concepts and theories to clinical situations, solve clinical problems, arrive at carefully thought-out decisions, and engage in critical thinking about these problems and solutions are essential competencies gained through clinical practice. Case method, case study, and grand rounds are appropriate teaching methods to help students meet these learning outcomes. Case method and case study describe a clinical situation developed around an actual or a hypothetical patient for student review and critique. In case method the case provided for analysis is generally shorter and more specific than in case study. Case studies are more comprehensive in nature, thereby presenting a complete picture of the patient and clinical situation. Grand rounds involve the observation and, often, interview of a patient or patients in a clinical setting or through a Web cast or multimedia program.

Each of these clinical teaching methods can be developed for students to apply concepts and theories to practice situations, identify actual and potential problems and propose varied approaches for solving them, weigh different decisions possible, and arrive at judgments as to the effectiveness of interventions. Case method and study and grand rounds provide experience for students in thinking through different clinical situations to gain a perspective of patients, families, and communities for whom they may be responsible in future practice.

SKILL IN PROBLEM SOLVING

There are varied perspectives of problem solving, decision making, and critical thinking. In general, *problem solving* is the ability to solve clinical problems, some relating to the patient and others that arise from clinical practice. Problem solving begins with recognizing and defining the problem, gathering data to clarify it further, developing solutions, and evaluating the effectiveness of potential solutions (Oermann & Gaberson, 2006).

Viewed as a cognitive *skill*, problem solving can be developed through repeated experiences with actual patients, such as in grand rounds, or through simulations provided by case method and study. The student does not need to give hands-on care to develop problem-solving skills. Observing and discussing the patient during grand rounds and analyzing cases provide essential experience in problem solving. These methods give students a perspective of what to expect in an actual clinical situation, typical problems the client may experience, interventions that should be considered for care, and similarities and differences across clinical situations.

SKILL IN DECISION MAKING

Case method and study and grand rounds also assist students in developing decision-making skills. *Decision making* involves considering different alternatives, weighing the consequences of each, and then arriving at a decision or choice as to the best alternative for the situation. With case method and study, clinical situations may be described that require a decision. Questions that accompany the case ask students to consider the alternatives possible and consequences of each, and then arrive at a decision following this analysis.

SKILL IN CRITICAL THINKING

Critical thinking enables the nurse to make reasoned and informed judgments in the practice setting and decide what to do in a given situation. Alfaro-LeFevre (2004) described *critical thinking* as purposeful and informed reasoning in clinical practice and in other settings. Critical thinking is results oriented: What are the results you need and what problems or issues must be addressed to achieve them? (Alfaro-LeFevre, p. 5). Critical thinking is reflective thinking about patient problems when the problem is not obvious or when the nurse knows what is wrong but is unsure what to do.

Through critical thinking the learner

- considers multiple perspectives to care,
- critiques different approaches possible in a clinical situation,
- arrives at judgments after considering multiple possibilities,
- raises questions about issues to clarify them further,
- resolves issues with a well-thought-out approach (Alfaro-LeFevre, 2004; Oermann, 1997, 1998; Oermann & Gaberson, 2006; Oermann, Truesdell, & Ziolkowski, 2000).

Another perspective of critical thinking involves its use in problem solving and decision making. Through critical thinking, students differentiate relevant from irrelevant data, identify cues in data and cluster them, propose varied diagnoses that might be possible, and decide on additional data needed for determining the diagnosis. In terms of interventions, critical thinking enables students to compare different approaches to care, weigh alternatives, and decide on the best approach considering these possibilities. The ability to think critically is essential for effective clinical practice.

CASE METHOD AND STUDY

Case method and case study serve similar purposes in clinical teaching: they provide a simulated case for student review and critique. In case method the case provided for analysis is generally shorter and more specific than in case study.

Case Method

In case method, short cases are developed around actual or hypothetical patients followed by open-ended questions to encourage students' thinking about the case. Depending on how the case is written, case method is effective for applying concepts and theories to clinical practice and for promoting problem solving, decision making, and critical thinking. Case method is a useful strategy for assisting students to learn how to analyze a case, identify problems and solutions, compare alternate decisions possible, and arrive at conclusions about different aspects of patient care (Oermann & Gaberson, 2006). It also assists students in relating course content to clinical practice and integrating different concepts and theories in a particular client situation. Examples of the case method teaching strategy are presented in Table 11.1.

TABLE 11.1   Case Method Examples

Problem Solving

Mrs. F has moderate dementia. She lets the nurse practitioner (NP) do a pelvic examination because she has a "woman's problem." The examination shows an anterior wall prolapse. While helping Mrs. F to get dressed, the NP observes that as soon as the patient stands up, urine begins leaking onto the floor. Mrs. F appears embarrassed.

1. List and prioritize Mrs. F's problems. Provide a rationale for how the problems are prioritized.
2. Develop a plan of care for Mrs. F.

Your patient is admitted from the Emergency Department with severe headache, right-sided weakness, and aphasia. Her temperature is normal, pulse 120, respirations 16, and blood pressure 180/120.

1. What are possible reasons for these symptoms? Provide an explanation for your answer.
2. What additional data would you collect on admission to your unit? Why is this information important to planning the patient's care?

You are working in a pediatrician's office. Mrs. C brings her son in for a check-up after a severe asthma attack a month ago that required emergency care. When you ask Mrs. C how her son is doing, she begins to cry softly. She tells you she is worried about his having another asthma attack and this time not recovering from it. When the pediatrician enters the examination room, Mrs. C is still crying. The physician says, "What's wrong? Look at him. He's doing great."

1. What would you say to Mrs. C, if anything, in this situation?
2. What would you say to the pediatrician, if anything?

You have a new patient, 81 years old, with congestive heart failure. The referral to your home health agency indicates that Mr. A has difficulty breathing, tires easily, and has edema in both legs making it difficult for him to get around. He lives alone.

1. What are patient problems you anticipate for Mr. A? Include a rationale for each of these problems.

At your first home visit, you find Mr. A sitting in a chair with his feet on the floor. During your assessment, he gets short of breath talking with you and has to stop periodically to catch his breath.

1. Describe at least three different nursing interventions that could be used in Mr. A's care.
2. Specify outcome criteria for evaluating the effectiveness of the interventions you selected.

TABLE 11.1   (Continued)

3. What would you teach Mr. A?
4. Identify one published research study that relates to Mr. A's care. Critique the study and describe whether or not you could use the findings in caring for Mr. A and similar patients.

Decision Making

Mrs. M is a 42-year-old elementary school teacher with a history of inflammatory bowel disease. She calls the clinic for an appointment because of diarrhea that has lasted for 2 weeks. The nurse answering the phone tells Mrs. M to stop taking all of her medications until she is seen in the clinic.

1. Do you agree or disagree with the nurse's advice to Mrs. M? Why?

You have been working in the clinical agency for nearly 6 months. Recently you noticed a colleague having difficulty completing his assignments on time. He also has been late for work on at least three occasions. Today you see him move from one patient to the next without washing his hands.

1. What are your options in this situation?
2. Discuss possible consequences of each option.
3. What would you do? Why is this the best approach?

Your patient has had diarrhea and abdominal pain for 8 days. She is scheduled for a number of diagnostic tests. As you complete her health history, she asks to see her chart.

1. What would you say to this patient?
2. What principles guide your decision? Provide a rationale for your response.

Mrs. J brings her 8-year-old daughter, Laura, into the office for her annual visit. In reviewing the immunization record, the nurse notices that Laura never received the second dose of MMR (measles, mumps, rubella). The nurse tells the mother not to worry. Laura can get the second dose when she is 11 or 12 years old.

1. Do you agree or disagree with the RN's advice to the mother? Provide a rationale for your decision.

Critical Thinking

Read the following statements: One in three adults and one in five adolescents are overweight. Being overweight is prevalent among certain racial and ethnic groups.

1. What additional information do you need before identifying the implications of this statement for your community?
2. Why is this information important?

(continues)

TABLE 11.1   Case Method Examples (Continued)

Mr. J is developmentally delayed but has been able to live alone with the help of a neighbor. The neighbor, however, is moving. The neighbor calls your clinic and asks if someone can help Mr. J.

1. What are your options in this situation?
2. What critical information is needed before you decide what to do?

The heart failure clinic at your hospital has been effective in reducing the number of readmissions, but to save costs, the hospital is closing it. As the nurse practitioner in that clinic, write a report as to why the clinic should remain open, with data to support your position. To whom would you send that report and why? Then write a report from the perspective of the hospital administration supporting closure of the clinic.

"Every American should have access to high quality and affordable health care."

1. Do you agree or disagree with that statement? Provide a rationale that supports your answer. Use at least two research studies to develop your rationale.
2. Then write a paper on the opposite perspective, using two other research studies for support of your ideas.

Case Study

A case study provides an actual patient situation or a hypothetical one for students to analyze and arrive at varied decisions. Case studies typically are longer and more comprehensive than in case method, providing background data about the patient, family history, and other information for a more complete picture. For this reason, students can analyze case studies in greater depth than with case method and present a more detailed rationale for their analysis. In their critique of the case study, students can describe the concepts and theories that guided their analysis, how they used them in understanding the case, and the literature they reviewed. A case study example is presented in Table 11.2.

Using Case Method and Case Study in Clinical Courses

Short cases, as in case method, and longer case studies can be integrated in clinical courses throughout the curriculum to assist students in applying concepts and theories to patient situations of increasing complexity. In beginning clinical courses, teachers can develop cases that present problems that are relatively easy to identify

TABLE 11.2 Case Study Example

Mary, 44 years old, is seen in the physician's office with hoarseness and a slight cough. During the assessment, Mary tells the nurse that she also has shortness of breath, particularly when walking fast and going up the stairs. Mary has never smoked. Her vital signs are:

BP	120/80
HR	88 bpm
Respirations	32/minute
Temperature	36.6°C (97.8°F)

Mary is married with two teenage daughters. She works part time as a substitute teacher. Mary has always been health conscious, watching her weight and eating properly. She tells the nurse how worried she is because she has read about women getting lung cancer even if they never smoked.

1. The physician orders a combined PET/CT scan. What is a PET/CT scan, and why was it ordered for Mary?
2. What would you say to Mary prior to the scan to prepare her for it?

A few weeks later Mary is diagnosed with lung adenocarcinoma.

1. What treatments are used for this type of cancer?
2. Select one of those treatments, explain what it is, and describe the standard nursing care for patients receiving it.
3. Add data about Mary and her family to the case. Modify your care plan to reflect Mary's individual needs at this time.
4. What resources are available in your community for Mary?

It is now 3 months after the initial diagnosis. Finish this case study by describing Mary's condition and your nursing care for her.

and require standard nursing interventions. At this level students learn how to apply concepts to clinical situations and think them through. Students can work as a group to analyze these cases, explore different perspectives of the clinical problem, and discuss possible approaches to use.

In the beginning, the teacher should think aloud and guide students through the analysis, pointing out significant cues in the case that would influence decision making. By thinking aloud, the teacher can model critical thinking step-by-step through a case. As students progress through the curriculum, the cases can become more complex with varied problems and approaches that could be used in the situation.

As part of the case analysis, Bentley (2001) suggested recording "What is Known" and "What is Unknown." The unknown information provides a basis for student learning in clinical practice. In Bentley's strategy, students locate the information through varied resources and later present the information and how they found it. This strategy can be implemented in pre- and postclinical conferences and can also be used in an online course. Students can analyze the cases online either individually or in small groups, including resources they used to better understand the case. Further discussion about the case can occur with the clinical group as a whole, or students can individually post their thoughts and reactions. Case studies analyzed in online courses are ideal for encouraging group work and collaborative learning (Halstead, 2005).

Case method and study can be used in many ways in a course. Cases can be analyzed individually or as a clinical group, in a conference setting or as an out-of-class activity. Based on the questions asked about the case, they can be used to meet many different learning outcomes of a clinical course. While they are effective as an instructional method, they can also be used for student evaluation and grading.

Complexity of Cases for Review.   Cases for review and critique may be of varying levels of complexity. Some cases may be designed with the problems readily apparent. Such cases describe the problem clearly and include sufficient information to guide decisions on how to intervene. Nitko (2004) called these cases "well-structured," providing an opportunity for students to apply concepts to a patient situation and develop an understanding of how they are used in clinical practice. Cases of this type link knowledge presented in class and through readings to practice situations. With well-structured cases there usually is one correct answer that students can identify based on what they are currently learning in the clinical course.

These cases are effective for students beginning a clinical course in which they have limited background and expertise. With well-structured cases, students can learn how to apply the concepts they are learning about in class and in their readings to clinical scenarios and explore patient problems in those scenarios. Well-structured cases give students an opportunity to practice their problem solving, decision making, and critical thinking before caring for an actual patient. Nitko (2004) suggested that with well-structured problems students can rehearse algorithms and procedures for solving problems (p. 208).

Most patient care situations, however, are not that easily solved. In clinical practice the problems sometimes are difficult to identify, or the nurse may be confident as to the patient's problem but unsure how to intervene. These are problems in Schön's (1990) "swampy lowland," ones that do not lend themselves to resolution by a technical and rational approach. These are cases that vary from the way the problems and solutions were presented in class and through readings. For cases such as these, the principles learned in class may not readily apply, and critical thinking is required for analysis and resolution.

Nitko (2004) referred to these cases as "ill-structured," describing problems that reflect real-life clinical situations faced by students. With ill-structured cases, different problems may be possible, there may be an incomplete data set to determine the problem, or the problem may be clear but multiple solutions may be possible. Table 11.3 presents examples of a well-structured and an ill-structured case.

Developing Cases

Case Components.   Case method and study have two components: a case *description* for review and analysis by the student and *questions* to answer about the case or its analysis. In case method, the situations described are typically short and geared to specific objectives to be met. Case studies include background information about the patient, family history, and complete assessment data to provide a comprehensive description of the patient or clinical situation.

The case should provide enough information for analysis without directing the students' thinking in a particular direction. The case may be developed first, then the questions, or the teacher may draft the questions first, then develop the case to present the clinical situation. Once students have experience in analyzing cases, another strategy is for students to develop a case scenario based on data provided by the teacher. In this method, students need to think about what diagnoses and patient problems might fit the data, which promotes their critical thinking.

The questions developed for a specific case are the key to its effective use. The questions should be geared to the outcomes to be met. For instance, if the intent of the case method or study is for students to analyze laboratory data, apply physiological principles, and use concepts of pathophysiology for the analysis, then the questions need to relate to each of these areas. Similarly, if the goal is to improve problem-solving skill, then the questions should ask about problems described in the case, alternate problems possible, supporting data, additional data needed, and varied solutions. With most cases, questions should be included that focus on the underlying thought process used to arrive at an answer rather than on the answer alone.

In designing cases to promote problem solving, the teacher should develop a case that asks students to

- identify patient and other problems apparent in the case,

- suggest alternate problems that might be possible if more information were available and identify the information needed,

TABLE 11.3   Well-Structured and Ill-Structured Cases

Well-Structured Case

Mrs. D, 53 years old, reports having bad headaches for the last month. The headaches occur about twice weekly, usually in the late morning. Initially the pain began as a throbbing at her right temple. Her headaches now affect either her right or left eye and temple. The pain is so severe, she usually goes to bed. Mrs. D reports that her neck hurts, and the nurse notes tenderness in the posterior neck on palpation.

1. What type or types of headache might Mrs. D be experiencing?
2. Describe additional data that should be collected from Mrs. D. Why is this information important to deciding what is wrong with Mrs. D?
3. Select two interventions that might be used for Mrs. D. Provide evidence for their use.

Ill-Structured Case

Ms. J, 35 years old, calls for an appointment because she fell yesterday at home. She has a few bruises from her fall and a "tingling feeling" in her legs. Ms. J had been at the eye doctor's last week for double vision.

1. What additional data should be collected from Ms. J? Why are these data important?
2. List laboratory and diagnostic tests for Ms. J. Why should these be ordered?
3. What are possible diagnoses to be considered for Ms. J?

- identify relevant and irrelevant information in the case,

- propose different approaches that might be used,

- identify advantages and disadvantages of each approach,

- select the best approaches for solving problems in the case situation,

- provide a theoretical rationale for these approaches,

- identify gaps in the literature and research as related to the case,

- evaluate the effectiveness of interventions,

- plan alternate interventions based on analysis of the case.

Problem-Solving Case Example

Ms. G, a 56-year-old patient admitted for shortness of breath and chest pain, is scheduled for a cardiac catheterization. She has been crying on and off for the last hour. When the nurse attempts to talk to her, Ms. G says, "Don't worry about me. I'm just tired."

1.   What is one problem in this situation that needs to be solved?

2.   What assumptions about Ms. G did you make in identifying this problem?

3.   What additional information would you collect from the patient and her medical records before intervening? Why is this information important?

Cases for decision making may be developed in two ways. The case may present a clinical situation up to the point of a decision, then ask students to critique the case and arrive at a decision. Or the case may describe a situation and decision, then ask whether students agree or disagree with it. For both of these types, the questions should lead the students through the decision-making process, and students should include a rationale for their responses.

For decision making, the teacher should develop a case that asks students to

- identify the decisions needed in the case,

- identify information in the case that is critical for arriving at a decision,

- specify additional data needed for a decision,

- examine alternative decisions possible and the consequences of each,

- arrive at a decision and provide a rationale for it.

Decision-Making Case Example

The charge nurse on the midnight shift in a large hospital assigns a nurse new to the unit to work with Ms. P, an experienced RN. Ms. P, however, is irate that she needs to orient a new nurse when she is so busy herself. Ms. P tells the new nurse that she is too busy to work with her tonight. When learning this, the charge nurse reassigns the new nurse to another RN.

1.   Do you agree or disagree with the charge nurse's decision? Why?

2.   Describe at least two strategies you could use in this situation. What are advantages and disadvantages of each?

3.   How would you handle this situation?

Case method and case study also meet critical thinking outcomes. There are a number of strategies that teachers can use when developing cases that are intended for critical thinking. These are listed in Table 11.4.

Critical-Thinking Case Example

You are a nurse practitioner working in a middle school. S, a 16-year-old, comes to your office for nausea and vomiting. She feels "bloated." She confides in you that she is pregnant and asks you not to tell her parents.

TABLE 11.4 Strategies for Developing Case Studies for Critical Thinking

Develop cases that:	Ask students to:
Present an issue for analysis, a question to be answered that has multiple possibilities, or a complex problem to be solved.	Analyze the case and provide a rationale for the thinking process they used for the analysis.
	Examine the assumptions underlying their thinking.
	Describe the evidence on which their reasoning was based.
	Describe the concepts and theories they used for their analysis and how they applied to the case.
Have different and conflicting points of view.	Analyze the case from their own point of view and then analyze the case from a different point of view.
Present complex data for analysis.	Analyze the data and draw possible inferences given the data.
	Specify additional information needed and why it is important.
Present clinical situations that are unique and offer different perspectives.	Analyze the situation, identify multiple perspectives possible, and examine assumptions made about the situation that influenced thinking.
Describe ethical issues and dilemmas.	Propose alternative solutions and consequences of different approaches.
	Weigh alternatives and arrive at a decision.
	Critique an issue from a different point of view.

1. What are your options at this time?
2. What option would you choose to implement? Why?
3. Choose another option that you listed for question 1. What are advantages and disadvantages of that approach over your first option?

Types of Questions With Case.   The questions are the key to effective use of the case method and study. The nursing process provides a framework for writing these questions. Students can be asked about data to collect, priority information needed, significant and insignificant data in the case, and other questions on assessment. They can be asked to list and prioritize current and potential patient problems, with a rationale. Questions can be directed at interventions and their evidence and at how students would decide on the best intervention for the patient. Lastly, questions can be directed toward outcomes to be evaluated in the case.

A case may be geared to one only phase of the nursing process, for example, including questions on interventions only, or to reflect other aspects of nursing care for the patient described in the case. The following case has a focus on assessment and identifying potential patient problems:

> Mrs. B, 29 years old, is seen for her prenatal checkup. She is in her 24th week of pregnancy. The nurse practitioner notes swelling of the ankles and around Mrs. B's eyes. Mrs. B has not been able to wear her rings for a week because of swelling. Her blood pressure is 144/96.

1. What are possible problems Mrs. B might be facing? List all possible problems given the available information.
2. What additional data should be collected at this time? Why?

Alternatively, the same case might be used to guide students in thinking about assumptions they make in patient care and the influence of those assumptions on their decision making. For this learning outcome, using the same case, the questions might be:

1. Name one possible problem for Mrs. B.
2. What assumptions did you make about Mrs. B's condition that led you to this problem?
3. List three actions to be taken at this time. Why is each of these important in Mrs. B's care? What thought process did you use to decide on these actions?
4. What would you do first? Why?

Unfolding Cases

A variation of case study is unfolding cases in which the clinical situation is ever-changing, thereby creating a simulation for students to critique. Glendon and Ulrich (1997) proposed writing three paragraphs. The first paragraph sets the context of the case, including background information about the patient and others, a description of the clinical situation, and questions for discussion by students. After the initial analysis of the case by the students, the next paragraph is revealed, changing the scenario in some way. Students then critique the new information and answer related questions. After reading the last paragraph, students complete a reflective writing exercise in which they project future learning needs and share individual feelings and reactions to the case. Unfolding cases also can be used in staff development (Ulrich & Glendon, 2002).

GRAND ROUNDS

Grand rounds involve the observation and, often, interview of a patient or several patients in the clinical setting, a Web cast of grand rounds conducted elsewhere, or a multimedia program of the grand rounds. Grand rounds provide an opportunity to observe a patient with a specific condition, discuss assessment and diagnoses, and propose interventions and changes in the plan of care. Rounds are valuable for examining issues facing patients and families and exposing students to situations they may not encounter in their own clinical experiences. Grand rounds may involve nursing students and staff members only or be interdisciplinary. Nursing grand rounds can also be used for staff education. Lannon (2005) described how grand rounds were developed as a means of providing staff nurses with a forum in which to share their clinical expertise and best practices with other staff.

Rather than conducting rounds in the clinical setting, faculty members may decide to use available Web casts of grand rounds. For example, Public Health Grand Rounds is a series of satellite broadcasts and Web casts that present case studies on public health issues (North Carolina Institute for Public Health, 2006). These would be valuable for use in a community health nursing course.

There are also CD-ROMs and other multimedia programs on grand rounds, which could be integrated in a clinical course. For example, Cincinnati Children's Hospital Medical Center provides Nursing Grand Rounds via streaming media (2006). Its Web site provides a list of current and archived grand rounds with active links to each program. Epstein and colleagues (2003) implemented two video projects, one of which was nursing grand rounds, to promote active student involvement in the classroom. Students in clinical groups were assigned to a specific patient problem related to course content such as care of patients with heart failure.

Students then role-played a patient, a staff nurse, an advanced practice nurse, a pharmacist, a physician, and other roles depending on the patient's diagnosis. The rounds were videotaped for students to review. The grand rounds promoted student learning about characteristics of common health problems, teamwork, and students' development of presentation skills (Epstein et al., 2003).

Grand rounds enable students to

- identify patient problems and issues in a clinical situation,

- evaluate the effectiveness of nursing and interdisciplinary interventions,

- share clinical knowledge with peers and identify gaps in their own understanding,

- develop new perspectives about the patient's care,

- gain insight into other ways of meeting patient needs,

- think critically about the nursing care they provide and that given by their peers,

- dialogue about patient care and changes in clinical practice with peers and experts participating in the rounds.

Sedlak and Doheny (2004) described a clinical teaching strategy that uses peer review during student-led rounds to promote critical thinking. At the end of each clinical day, groups of three to four students each conduct walking rounds in place of a postclinical conference. Students briefly describe important physical and psychosocial assessment data, nursing diagnoses, interventions, and outcomes while other students listen. They then introduce their patients to the group of students, if possible. After leaving the patient's room, students ask questions and discuss the patient's care, identifying areas needing further clarification.

Regardless of whether the rounds are conducted in the clinical setting or viewed on a Web cast or videotape, the teacher should first identify the outcomes that students should meet at the end of the rounds. The outcomes guide the teacher in planning the rounds and their focus. Second, it should be clear why the particular patient or clinical situation was selected for grand rounds. Third, the questions asked after rounds should encourage students to think critically about the patient and care, compare this case to the textbook picture and other patients for whom students have cared, and explore alternate interventions and perspectives of the situation. The final area of discussion should focus on what students have learned from this experience and new insights they have gained about clinical practice. Students might write a short paper reflecting on their learning and new perspectives.

Grand rounds may be conducted by an advanced practice nurse, a staff nurse, the teacher, a student, or another health professional. For student-led rounds, the teacher is responsible for confirming the plan with the patient. Patients should be assured of their right to refuse participation and should be comfortable to tell those involved in the rounds when they no longer want to continue with it.

For grand rounds in the clinical setting, activities at the patient's bedside should begin with an introduction of the patient to the students, emphasizing the patient's contribution to student learning. If possible, the person conducting the rounds should include the patient and family in the discussion, seeking their perspective of the health problem and input into care. The teacher's role is that of consultant, clarifying information and assisting the student in keeping the discussion on the goals set for the rounds. Students should direct any questions to the teacher prior to and after the grand rounds, and sensitive issues should be discussed when the rounds are completed and out of the patient's presence.

SUMMARY

Case method and case study describe a clinical situation developed around an actual or a hypothetical patient for student review and critique. In case method, the case provided for analysis is generally shorter and more specific than in case study. Case studies are more comprehensive in nature, thereby presenting a complete picture of the patient and clinical situation.

With these clinical teaching methods, students apply concepts and theories to practice situations, identify actual and potential problems and propose varied approaches for solving them, weigh different decisions possible, and arrive at judgments as to the effectiveness of interventions. As such, case method and study provide experience for students in thinking through different clinical situations. They are valuable for promoting development of problem-solving, decision-making, and critical-thinking skills.

Grand rounds involve the observation of a patient or several patients in the clinical setting, in a Web cast, or in a multimedia program. Grand rounds may be conducted for nursing students and staff only or as an interdisciplinary activity. Rounds provide an opportunity to observe a patient with a specific condition, review assessment data, discuss interventions and their effectiveness, and make changes in the plan of care. Rounds are also valuable for examining issues facing patients and discussing ways of resolving them. Grand rounds, similar to case method and study, provide an opportunity for exploring patient problems and varied solutions, analyzing care and proposing new interventions, and gaining insight into different patient situations.

REFERENCES

Alfaro-LeFevre, R. (2004). *Critical thinking and clinical judgment* (3rd ed.). St. Louis: Saunders.

Bentley, G. W. (2001). Problem-based learning. In A. J. Lowenstein & M. J. Bradshaw, *Fuszard's innovative teaching strategies in nursing* (3rd ed., pp. 83–106). Gaithersburg, MD: Aspen.

Cincinnati Children's Hospital Medical Center. (2006). *Nursing grand rounds*. Retrieved March 8, 2006, from http://www.cincinnatichildrens.org/ed/cme/streaming-media/library/nursing/

Epstein, C. D., Hovancsek, M. T., Dolan, P. L., Durner, E., Rocco, N. L., Preiszig, P., et al. (2003). Lights! Camera! Action! Video projects in the classroom. *Journal of Nursing Education, 42*, 558–561.

Glendon, K., & Ulrich, D. L. (1997). Unfolding cases: An experiential learning model. *Nurse Educator, 22*, 15–18.

Halstead, J. A. (2005). Promoting critical thinking through online discussion. In M. H. Oermann & K. T. Heinrich (Eds.), *Annual review of nursing education* (Vol. 3, pp. 143–163). New York: Springer Publishing.

Lannon, S. L. (2005). Nursing grand rounds: Promoting excellence in nursing. *Journal for Nurses in Staff Development, 21*, 221–226.

Nitko, A. J. (2004). *Educational assessment of students* (4th ed.). Upper Saddle River, NJ: Pearson Prentice Hall.

North Carolina Institute for Public Health. (2006, February 13). *Public health grand rounds*. Retrieved March 8, 2006, from http://www.publichealthgrandrounds.unc.edu/

Oermann, M. H. (1997). Evaluating critical thinking in clinical practice. *Nurse Educator, 22*, 25–28.

Oermann, M. H. (1998). How to assess critical thinking in clinical practice. *Dimensions of Critical Care Nursing, 17*, 322–327.

Oermann, M. H., & Gaberson, K. B. (2006). *Evaluation and testing in nursing education* (2nd ed.). New York: Springer Publishing.

Oermann, M. H., Truesdell, S., & Ziolkowski, L. (2000). Strategy to assess, develop, and evaluate critical thinking. *Journal of Continuing Education in Nursing, 31*, 155–160.

Schön, D. A. (1990). *Educating the reflective practitioner*. San Francisco: Jossey-Bass.

Sedlak, C. A., & Doheny, M. O. (2004). Critical thinking: What's new and how to foster thinking among nursing students. In M. H. Oermann & K. T. Heinrich (Eds.), *Annual review of nursing education* (Vol. 2, pp. 185–204). New York: Springer Publishing.

Ulrich, D., & Glendon, K. (2002). Managers forum. Unfolding case study instruction. *Journal of Emergency Nursing, 28*, 246–247.

Chapter 12

Discussion and Clinical Conferences

Discussions with learners and clinical conferences provide a means of sharing information, developing problem-solving and critical-thinking skills, and learning how to collaborate with others in a group. Discussion is an exchange of ideas for a specific purpose; clinical conferences are a form of group discussion that focus on some aspect of clinical practice. Teachers and students engage in many discussions in planning, carrying out, and evaluating the clinical learning activities. Similarly, there are varied types of clinical conferences for use in teaching. Effective conferences and discussions require an understanding of their goals, the types of questions for encouraging exchange of ideas and higher level thinking, and the roles of the teacher and students.

DISCUSSION

Discussions between teacher and student, preceptor and orientee, and nurse manager and staff occur frequently but do not always promote learning. Often these discussions involve the teacher telling the learner what to do or not to do for a patient. Discussions, though, should be an exchange of ideas through which the teacher, by asking open-ended questions and supporting learner responses, encourages students to arrive at their own decisions or to engage in self-assessment about clinical practice. Discussions are not intended to be a presentation of the teacher's ideas to the students. In a discussion both teacher and student actively participate in sharing ideas and considering alternate perspectives.

Discussions give learners an opportunity to interact with one another, critique one another's ideas, and learn from others. For that reason, discussions are an effective method for promoting critical thinking. The teacher can ask open-ended and thought-provoking questions, which encourage critical thinking if students perceive that they are free to discuss their own ideas and those of others involved in the discussion. The teacher is a resource for students, giving immediate feedback and further instruction as needed. Discussions also provide a forum for students to explore feelings associated with their clinical practice, clarify values and ethical dilemmas, and learn to interact in a group format. Those outcomes are not as easily met in a large group setting. Over a period of time, discussions help students learn to collaborate with peers in working toward solving clinical problems.

Creating a Climate for Discussion

An important role of the teacher is to develop a climate in which students are comfortable discussing concepts and issues without fear that the ideas expressed will affect the teacher's evaluation of their performance and subsequent clinical grade. Similarly, discussions between preceptor and orientee and between manager and staff should be carried out in an atmosphere in which nurses feel comfortable to express their own opinions and ideas and to question others' assumptions. Discussions are for formative evaluation, not summative; they provide feedback to learners individually or in a small group to guide their learning and thinking. Without this climate for exchanging ideas, though, discussions cannot be carried out effectively because students fear that their comments may influence their clinical evaluation and grade, or for nurses, their performance ratings.

The teacher sets an atmosphere in which listening, respect for others' comments and ideas, and openness to new perspectives are valued. Learners need to be free to discuss their ideas with the teacher, who can guide their critical thinking through careful questioning. Without support from the teacher, students will not participate freely in the discussion nor will they be willing to examine controversial points of view, critique different perspectives of care and decisions, or share misunderstandings with the teacher and peers. To facilitate students' learning in the clinical setting, faculty members need to create an environment of mutual respect (Wolff, 2007).

Studies on teacher effectiveness highlight the importance of this interpersonal relationship between teacher and students. Conveying confidence in students and their ability to perform in clinical practice, demonstrating respect for students, being honest and direct with them, and encouraging students to ask questions and participate freely in discussions are important characteristics of effective clinical teaching. In a study by Gignac-Caille and Oermann (2001) of effective clinical teaching behaviors, the 10 most important characteristics identified by nursing faculty were related to teaching skills and developing positive interpersonal relationships with students. Considering the many demands on students as they learn to care for patients, students need to view the teacher as someone who supports them in their learning. Providing support to students is a critical role of clinical teachers (Manias & Aitken, 2005).

Guidelines for Discussion

Discussions may be carried out individually with learners or in a small group. The size of the group for a discussion can range from 2 to 10 people. Any larger group makes it difficult for each person to participate.

The teacher is responsible for planning the discussion to meet the intended outcomes of the clinical course or specific goals to be achieved through the discussion. An effective teacher keeps the discussion focused; avoids talking too much, with students in a passive role; and avoids sidetracking. While the teacher may initiate the discussion, the interaction needs to revolve around the students, not the teacher. Rephrasing students' questions for them to answer suggests that the teacher has confidence in students' ability to arrive at answers and provides opportunities to develop critical thinking skills. Open-ended questions without one specific answer encourage critical thinking among both students and nurses (Oermann, Truesdell, & Ziolkowski, 2000).

The teacher should also be aware of the environment in which the discussion takes place. Chairs should be arranged in a configuration, such as a circle, semicircle or U-shape, that encourages interaction. For some discussions, students may be divided into pairs or other smaller groups. Table 12.1 summarizes the roles of the teacher and students in clinical discussions.

Following are guidelines for planning a discussion and effectively using it in the clinical setting:

- Identify the outcomes and goals to be achieved in the discussion considering the time frame.

- Plan questions for structured discussions ahead of time. They may be written for the teacher only or also for students. If not written, the teacher should think about the questions to ask, their order, and important content to discuss prior to beginning the interaction.

- Plan *how* the discussion will be carried out. Will all students in the clinical group participate, or will they be divided into smaller groups or pairs, then share the results of their individual discussions to the clinical group?

- Sequence questions depending on the desired outcomes of the discussion.

TABLE 12.1   Roles of Teacher and Student in Discussion

Teacher

Plans discussion
Presents problem, issue, case for analysis
Develops questions for discussion
Facilitates discussion with students as active participants
Develops and maintains atmosphere for open discussion of ideas and issues
Keeps time
Avoids sidetracking
Provides feedback

Student

Prepares for discussion
Participates actively in discussion
Works collaboratively with group members to arrive at solutions and decisions
Examines different points of view
Is willing to modify own view and perspective to reach group consensus

Teacher and Student

Summarize outcomes of discussion
Relate discussion to theory and research
Identify implications of discussion for other clinical situations

---

- Ask open-ended questions that encourage multiple perspectives and different lines of thinking.

- Think about how the questions are phrased before asking them.

- Ask questions to the group as a whole or ask for volunteers to respond. If questions are directed to a specific learner, be sensitive to his or her comfort in responding and do not create undue stress for the student. If discomfort is obvious, the teacher should provide prompts or cues for responding.

- Wait 3 to 5 seconds or longer between the question and request for students to answer it (Brualdi, 1998).

- Give students *time* to answer the questions. If no one responds, the teacher should try rephrasing the question.

- Reinforce students' answers indicating why they were or were not appropriate for the question.

- Without overusing it, give nonverbal and verbal feedback to encourage student participation.

- Avoid interrupting the learner even if errors are noted in the line of thinking or information.

- Correct students' errors in thinking when they are finished answering the question. It is critical that the teacher give feedback to students and correct their errors without belittling them. The goal is to focus on the answer and errors in reasoning, not on the student.

- Listen carefully to students' responses and make notes to remember points made in the discussion. The teacher should tell students ahead of time that any notes are for use only during the discussion, not for student evaluation or other purposes. The notes should be destroyed so students are assured of their freedom to respond in discussions.

- Assess own skill in directing the discussions and identify areas for improvement.

Discussions may begin with questions raised by the teacher or by students, or discussions may be integrated with other instructional methods, such as case scenarios, simulations, games, role-play, and media clips. Case scenarios, for instance, may be critiqued and then discussed by students in a clinical conference. Or students may play a game and complete a role-play exercise, followed by discussion. Media clips provide an effective format for presenting a clinical situation for analysis and discussion.

Purposes of Discussion

In a discussion the teacher has an opportunity to ask carefully selected questions about students' thinking and the rationale used for arriving at decisions and positions about issues. Discussions promote several types of learning depending on the goals and structure:

- Developing the cognitive skills of problem solving, decision making, and critical thinking

- Debriefing clinical experiences

- Developing cooperative learning and group process skills

- Assessing own learning

- Developing oral communication skills

Every discussion will not necessarily promote each of these learning outcomes. The teacher should be clear as to the intent of the discussion so it may be geared to the particular outcomes to be achieved. For instance, discussions for critical thinking require carefully selected questions that examine alternate possibilities and what-if types of questions. This same type of questioning, however, may not be necessary if the goal is to develop cooperative learning or group process skills.

Developing Cognitive Skills.   An important purpose of discussion is to promote development of problem-solving, decision-making, and critical-thinking skills. Discussions are effective because they provide an opportunity for the teacher to gear the questioning toward each of these skills. Not all discussions, though, lead to these higher levels of thinking. The key is the type of question asked by the teacher or discussed among students—questions need to encourage students to examine alternate perspectives and points of view in a given situation and to provide a rationale for their thinking. Table 12.2 presents strategies for directing discussions toward development of higher level cognitive skills.

In these discussions, students can be given a hypothetical or real clinical situation involving a patient, family, or community to critique and identify potential problems. Students can then discuss possible decisions in that situation, consequences of different options they considered as part of their decision making, and other points of view. Case scenarios can be distributed to students prior

TABLE 12.2   Discussions for Cognitive Skill Development

Ask students to:

Identify problems and issues in a real or hypothetical clinical situation
Identify alternate problems possible
Assess the problem further
Differentiate relevant and irrelevant information for problem or issue being discussed
Discuss own point of view and those of others
Examine assumptions they made and those of other students
Identify different solutions, courses of action, and consequences of each
Consider both positive and negative consequences
Compare possible alternatives and defend why they would choose one particular solution
    or action over another
Take a position about an issue and provide a rationale both for and against that position
Identify their own biases, values, and beliefs that influence their thinking
Identify obstacles to solving a problem
Evaluate the effectiveness of interventions and approaches to solving problems

to discussion; students can then review related literature and locate other resources to help them analyze the case (Bentley, 2001). Discussions are particularly valuable in helping students analyze ethical dilemmas, consider different points of view, and explore their own values and beliefs.

Debriefing Clinical Experiences.   Discussions provide an opportunity for students to report on their clinical learning activities and describe and analyze the care they provided to patients, families, and communities. In these discussions students receive feedback from peers and the teacher about their clinical decisions and other possible approaches they could use with their patient's care. Debriefing also provides an opportunity to share feelings about clinical practice and develop support systems for students (Stokes & Kost, 2005). Issues with patients, staff, and others may be examined and critiqued by the group.

Debriefing clinical experiences allows students to share feelings and perceptions about their patients and clinical situations in a comfortable environment. Ward and Apsey (2000) recommended that in clinical conferences students should be free to share their individual experiences without the concern of being evaluated by the teacher.

Developing Cooperative Learning Skills.   Group discussions are effective for promoting cooperative learning skills. In cooperative learning students work in small groups to meet predetermined goals (Johnson & Johnson, 2003). Students are actively involved in their learning and fostering the learning of others in the group. Stiles (2006) emphasized that in cooperative learning, the success of the group of students who are working together depends on the success of each student in that group: Students are accountable for their own learning as well as how much each person in their group learns.

Discussions using cooperative learning strategies begin with the teacher planning the discussion, presenting a task to be completed by the group or a problem to be solved, developing an environment for open discussion, and facilitating the discussion. Students work cooperatively in groups to propose solutions, complete the task, and present the results of their discussions to the rest of the students. Students can work in pairs or small groups to avoid too large a group for discussion.

Assessing Own Learning.   Discussions provide a means for students to assess their own learning, identify gaps in their understanding, and learn from others in a non-threatening environment. Students can ask questions of the group and use the teacher and peers as resources for their learning. If the teacher is effective in developing an atmosphere for open discussion, students, in turn, will share their feelings, concerns, and questions as a beginning to their continued development.

Developing Oral Communication Skills.   Ability to present ideas orally, as well as in written form, is an important outcome to be achieved by students in clinical courses (O'Connor, 2006). Discussions provide experience for students in presenting ideas to a group, explaining concepts clearly, handling questions raised by others, and refining presentation style. Participation in a discussion requires formulating ideas and presenting them logically to the group.

Students may make formal presentations to the clinical group as a way of developing their oral communication skills. They may lead a discussion and present on a specific topic related to the outcomes of the clinical course. Discussion provides an opportunity for peers and the teacher to give feedback to students on how well students communicated their ideas to others and to improve their communication techniques. Deering and Eichelberger (2002) developed an innovative approach for improving students' communication abilities and gaining insight into their own communication styles. Using online discussions, small groups of 4 or 5 students each analyzed their communication styles, tried and practiced new communication techniques, and provided feedback to one another on their techniques.

Table 12.3 presents an evaluation form that students may use to rate the quality of presentations and provide feedback on ability to lead a group discussion. This

TABLE 12.3   Evaluation Form for Rating Presentations in Conferences

Name _____

Title of Presentation _____

Rate each of the behaviors listed below. Circle the appropriate number and give feedback to the presenter in the space provided.

Behavior	Rating				
	1 To a limited extent	2	3	4	5 To a great extent
Leadership Role in Conference					
1. Leads the group in discussion of ideas.	1	2	3	4	5
2. Encourages active participation of peers in conference.	1	2	3	4	5
3. Encourages open discussion of ideas.	1	2	3	4	5
4. Helps group synthesize ideas presented.	1	2	3	4	5

Comments:

TABLE 12.3 (Continued)

Quality of Content Presented

5. Prepares objectives for presentation that reflect clinical goals.	1	2	3	4	5
6. Presents content that relates to objectives and is relevant for students' clinical practice.	1	2	3	4	5
7. Presents content that is accurate and up-to-date.	1	2	3	4	5
8. Presents content that reflects theory and research.	1	2	3	4	5

Comments:

Quality of Presentation

9. Organizes and presents material logically.	1	2	3	4	5
10. Explains ideas clearly.	1	2	3	4	5
11. Plans presentation considering time demands and needs of clinical group.	1	2	3	4	5
12. Emphasizes key points.	1	2	3	4	5
13. Encourages students to ask questions.	1	2	3	4	5
14. Answers students' questions accurately.	1	2	3	4	5
15. Supports alternate viewpoints and encourages their discussion.	1	2	3	4	5
16. Is enthusiastic.	1	2	3	4	5

Comments:

form is not intended for summative or grading purposes, but instead is designed for giving feedback to students following a presentation to the clinical group.

Level of Questions

The level of questions asked in any discussion is the key to directing it toward the intended learning outcomes. In most clinical discussions the goal is to avoid a predominance of factual questions and focus instead on higher level and open-ended questions. Teachers can use a framework such as Bloom's taxonomy to sequence questions in a discussion or can level those questions in a more general way, beginning with recall (low level) and progressing through clarifying to critical thinking (high level).

The taxonomy of the cognitive domain, related to knowledge and intellectual skills, was developed by Bloom (Bloom, Englehart, Furst, Hill, & Krathwohl, 1956) many years ago but is still of value today for developing test items and for leveling questions. Learning in the cognitive domain includes the acquisition of facts and specific information, concepts and theories, and higher level cognitive skills (Oermann & Gaberson, 2006). The cognitive taxonomy includes six levels that increase in complexity: knowledge, comprehension, application, analysis, synthesis, and evaluation. Because these levels are arranged in a hierarchy, recall of specific facts and information is the least complex level of learning and evaluating clinical situations and making judgments, the most complex.

The cognitive taxonomy is useful in asking questions in a discussion or planning questions for student response because it levels them along a continuum from ones requiring only recall of facts to higher level questions requiring synthesis of knowledge and evaluation. The teacher may begin by asking students factual questions and then progress to questions that are answered based on comprehension and understanding of the facts, the application of concepts and theories to clinical practice, analysis, synthesis of material from different sources, and evaluation.

A description and sample questions for each of the six levels of the cognitive taxonomy follow. Sample words for use in developing questions at each level are presented in Table 12.4.

1. Knowledge: Recall of facts and specific information; memorization of facts.
    "Define the term percussion."
    "What is this type of dysrhythmia called?"
2. Comprehension: Understanding; ability to describe and explain.
    "Tell me about your patient's shortness of breath."
    "What does this potassium level indicate?"
3. Application: Use of information in a *new* or *novel* situation; ability to use knowledge in a new situation.
    "Why are these interventions the most effective ones for your patient?"
    "Tell me about your patient's problems and related pathophysiological changes. Why are each of these changes important for you to monitor?"

TABLE 12.4   Question Classification With Sample Words for Questions

Level	Types of Question	Sample Words for Questions
1. Knowledge	*Recall:* Questions that can be answered by recall of facts and previously learned information	Define, identify, list, name, recall
2. Comprehension	*Understand:* Questions that can be answered by explaining and describing	Describe, differentiate, draw conclusions, explain, give examples of, interpret, tell me in your own words
3. Application	*Use:* Questions that require use of information in new situations	Apply, relate, use
4. Analysis	*Divide into component parts:* Questions that ask student to break down material into its component parts, to analyze data and clinical situations	Analyze, compare, contrast, detect, identify reasons and assumptions, provide evidence to support conclusions, relate
5. Synthesis	*Develop new ideas and products:* Questions or directives that ask students to develop new ideas, plans, products	Construct, create, design, develop, propose a plan, suggest a new approach
6. Evaluation	*Evaluate:* Questions that require student to make a judgment based on criteria	Appraise, assess, critique, evaluate, judge, select on basis of

4.   Analysis: Ability to break down material into component parts and identify the relationships among them.

"What effects does the organizational structure of the hospital and its home care agency have on services for patients and your role as a nurse?"

"What assumptions did you make about this family that influenced your decisions? What are alternate approaches to consider?"

5.   Synthesis: Ability to develop new ideas and materials; combining elements to form a new product.

"Tell me about your plan to improve prenatal care for the women who come to your clinic. Why is your plan better than the existing services?"

"Develop a care plan for patients receiving home care after hip replacement."

6. Evaluation: Judgments about value based on internal and external criteria; evaluating extent to which materials meet predetermined criteria.

    "Take a position for or against closing the clinic and shifting patients to the other center. Provide a rationale for your position."

    "What is the impact on patients and families of providing one less home care visit?"

Questions for discussions should be sequenced from low to high level. The taxonomy provides a schema for asking progressively higher level questions (Profetto-McGrath, Smith, Day, & Yonge, 2004; Wink, 1993). These higher level questions cannot be answered by memory alone and often have more than one answer. Higher level questions ask students to apply information they have learned to patient care or a clinical scenario, analyze a complex clinical situation, synthesize content, or evaluate options and alternates (Mertler, 2003; Oermann, 2004).

An example of a progression of questions using the taxonomy follows:

Knowledge: "Define the gate control theory of pain."

Comprehension: "Explain the physiological mechanisms underlying the gate control theory of pain."

Application: "Tell me about an intervention you are using for your patient and how its use and effectiveness may be explained by the gate control theory."

Analysis: "Your patient seems more agitated near the end of the shift. What additional data have you collected? What are possible reasons for this response?"

Synthesis: "Develop a pain management plan for your patient now and for his discharge home."

Evaluation: "You indicated that your patient's pain continues to increase. What alternate pain interventions do you propose? Why would these interventions be more effective?"

Research suggests that teachers by nature do not ask high level questions of students. Typically the questions asked in a discussion tend to focus on recall and comprehension rather than higher levels of thinking (Craig & Page, 1981; Phillips & Duke, 2001; Profetto-McGrath et al., 2004; Sellappah, Hussey, Blackmore, & McMurray, 1998; Wang & Blumberg, 1983; Wink, 1995). While the intent of clinical discussions may be to improve analytical thinking, this goal will not be met with questions that are answered by memorization of facts and specific information. Careful questioning with attention to using cognitively high level questions encourages students to answer at high levels and think critically (Profetto-McGrath et al., 2004, p. 364).

Rossignol (2000) recommended that faculty members monitor the level of questions they ask in their interactions with students. In this study of 30 post-clinical conferences, only one fourth of the interactions were at a high cognitive level. However, faculty members encouraged students' participation and had positive interactions with them.

Socratic Method

The Socratic method may also be used as a basis for discussion. Socratic questions raise issues for students to consider, require analytical thinking to respond, and promote critical thinking. Socratic thinking allows the student to form connections among ideas (Elder & Paul, 2002). Socratic questions are an effective strategy when students are puzzled about a patient's problem and approaches to use or are faced with a problematic area of thinking.

Paul (1993, p. 336) identified seven aims of Socratic questioning:

1. Raise basic issues.
2. Probe beneath the surface.
3. Pursue problematic areas of thought.
4. Discover structure of own thinking.
5. Develop sensitivity to clarity, accuracy, and relevance.
6. Arrive at judgments through own reasoning.
7. Identify claims, evidence, conclusions, questions-at-issue, assumptions, implications, and different points of view.

Socratic questions are open-ended, with multiple responses possible. The questions ask students to consider different alternatives and varied points of view and to defend their choices. Usually, no one answer is correct. After exploring these answers with students, the teacher can ask them to make connections to other clinical scenarios and to generalize learning from one patient and clinical situation to others. Examples of connecting questions are

- "How is your assessment of Ms. J similar to the patient you cared for last week with the same diagnosis?"

- "What patterns do you find in the data?"

- "What are similarities in nursing interventions for Mrs. P and what you learned about in class? In what ways does your nursing care differ and why?"

One outcome of this line of questioning is to increase students' understanding of difficult concepts by having them arrive at a general understanding of a problem and solution that is applicable to other possible clinical scenarios (Oermann, 1997).

Another model for using Socratic questions in a discussion is based on a taxonomy by Paul (1993). This model suggests different types of questions a teacher can ask to encourage critical thinking:

- Questions of clarification,

- Questions that probe assumptions,

- Questions that probe reasons and evidence,

- Questions about differing viewpoints or perspectives,

- Questions that probe implications and consequences (Elder & Paul, 2002; Paul, 1993).

Table 12.5 provides sample questions in each category that the teacher might use in clinical discussions.

CLINICAL CONFERENCES

Clinical conferences are discussions in which students share information about their clinical experiences, engage in critical thinking about clinical practice, lead others in discussions, and give formal presentations to the group. Some clinical conferences involve other disciplines and provide opportunities to work with other health care professionals in planning and evaluating patient care. Conferences serve the same goals as any discussion: developing problem-solving, decision-making, and critical-thinking skills; debriefing clinical experiences; developing cooperative learning and group process skills; assessing own learning; and developing oral communication skills. Guidelines for conducting clinical conferences are the same as for discussion and therefore are not repeated here.

TABLE 12.5   Socratic Questions

Clarification Questions

- Tell me about your patient—what is his/her primary problem?
- Of all your patient's problems, what is the most important one? Why?
- Explain what you mean by _____.

Questions to Probe Assumptions

- Tell me one decision you made today for your patient. Why did you decide on that?
- You appear to be assuming that _____. Why did you make that assumption?
- What assumptions did you make about this patient? Is that always true?

Questions to Probe Reasons

- What are possible reasons for _____?
- Why do you think _____?
- What evidence did you use to guide your thinking?

Questions on Differing Perspectives

- What are other possible interpretations? Perspectives?
- What are alternate approaches that might be used? Why might these be as or more effective than your interventions?
- Tell me one other way of interpreting this clinical situation.

Questions on Consequences

- What effect would _____ have on your patient?
- Tell me different approaches that could be used and possible results.
- Think about a decision you made today. Now tell me one alternative decision and its consequences.

Types of Conferences

There are many types of clinical conferences. *Preclinical conferences* are small group discussions that precede clinical learning activities. In preclinical conferences students ask questions about their clinical learning activities, seek clarification about their patients' care and other aspects of clinical practice, and share concerns with the teacher and with peers. Preclinical conferences assist students in identifying patient problems, setting priorities, and planning care; they prepare students for their clinical activities. An important role of the teacher in preclinical conferences is to assure that students have the essential knowledge and competencies to complete their clinical activities. In many instances the teacher needs to instruct students further and fill in the gaps in students' learning. Preclinical conferences may be conducted on a one-to-one basis with students or as a clinical group.

Postclinical conferences are held at the conclusion of clinical learning activities. Postclinical conferences provide a forum for analyzing patient care and exploring other options, thereby facilitating critical thinking. Postclinical conferences may be used for peer review and critiquing each other's work. They are not intended, however, as substitutes for classroom instruction with the teacher lecturing and presenting new content to students. A similar problem often occurs with guest speakers who treat the conference as a class, lecturing to students about their area of expertise rather than encouraging group discussion.

Clinical conferences can also focus on ethical and professional issues associated with clinical practice. Conferences of this type encourage critical thinking about issues that students have encountered or may encounter in the future. In these conferences students can analyze events that occurred in the clinical setting, ones in which they were personally involved or learned about through their clinical experience. A student can present the situation to the group for analysis and discussion. The discussion should focus on varied approaches that might be used and how to decide on the best strategy. What-if questions are effective for this type of conference.

Students and faculty alike are often fatigued at the end of the clinical practicum. To actively involve students in postclinical conferences, Glendon and Ulrich (2004) recommend simulations, role-play, storytelling, and writing exercises that the teacher connects to the learning experiences of students. Rather than each student sharing what he or she did in clinical practice, discussions that focus on higher level learning and critical thinking and that involve each student are more effective.

Debates provide a forum for analyzing problems and issues in depth, analyzing opposing viewpoints, and developing and defending a position to be taken. In a debate students should provide a rationale for their decisions. Debates developed around clinical issues give students an opportunity to prepare an argument for or against a particular position and to take a stand on an issue.

Setting for Clinical Conferences

Clinical conferences can be face-to-face in the clinical or academic setting, or they can be conducted online. Hamera and Wright (2004) evaluated the effectiveness of an online clinical conference for students enrolled in their advanced psychiatric mental health nursing course. In their online clinical conferences, students raised important issues about their practice and were involved in the discussions. One disadvantage identified by students was a lack of spontaneity compared to traditional face-to-face conferences.

In a study by Cooper, Taft, and Thelen (2004) comparing online and face-to-face clinical conferences, students reported that in online discussions they could participate more and that the conferences were more convenient. Students also reported that online conferences provided more opportunities to reflect on and discuss ethical issues. Students were able to achieve the outcomes of the clinical conferences through their online discussions.

SUMMARY

Discussions are an exchange of ideas in a small group format. They provide a forum for students to express ideas, explore feelings associated with their clinical practice, clarify values and ethical dilemmas, and learn to interact in a group format. Over a period of time, students learn to collaborate with peers in working toward solving clinical problems.

The teacher is a resource for students. By asking open-ended questions and supporting learner responses, the teacher encourages students to arrive at their own decisions and to engage in self-assessment about clinical practice. The teacher develops a climate in which students are comfortable discussing concepts and issues without fear that the ideas expressed will affect the teacher's evaluation of their performance and subsequent clinical grade.

Discussions promote several types of learning: developing problem-solving, decision-making, and critical-thinking skills; debriefing clinical experiences; developing cooperative learning and group process skills; assessing own learning; and developing oral communication skills. The level of questions asked in any discussion is the key to directing it toward the intended learning outcomes. In most clinical discussions the goal is to avoid a predominance of factual questions and focus instead on clarifying and higher level questions. Questions for student response may be leveled along a continuum from ones requiring only recall of facts to higher level questions requiring synthesis of knowledge and evaluation.

Clinical conferences are discussions in which students analyze patient care and clinical situations, lead others in discussions about clinical practice, present ideas in a group format, and give presentations to the group. Conferences serve the same goals as any discussion.

REFERENCES

Bentley, G. W. (2001). Problem-based learning. In A. J. Lowenstein & M. J. Bradshaw (Eds.), *Fuszard's innovative teaching strategies in nursing* (3rd ed., pp. 83–106). Gaithersburg, MD: Aspen.

Bloom, B. S., Englehart, M. D., Furst, E. J., Hill, W. H., & Krathwohl, D. R. (1956). *Taxonomy of educational objectives. The classification of educational goals. Handbook I: Cognitive domain.* White Plains, NY: Longman.

Brualdi, A. C. (1998). *Classroom questions.* Washington, DC: ERIC Clearinghouse on Assessment and Evaluation. (ERIC Document Reproduction Service No. ED422407)

Cooper, C., Taft, L. B., & Thelen, M. (2004). Examining the role of technology in learning: An evaluation of online clinical conferencing. *Journal of Professional Nursing, 20,* 160–166.

Craig, J. L., & Page, G. (1981). The questioning skills of nursing instructors. *Journal of Nursing Education, 20,* 18–23.

Deering, C. G., & Eichelberger, L. (2002). Mirror, mirror on the wall: Using online discussion groups to improve interpersonal skills. *CIN: Computers, Informatics, Nursing, 20,* 150–154.

Elder, L., & Paul, R. (2002). *The miniature guide to the art of asking essential questions.* Santa Rosa, CA: Foundation for Critical Thinking.

Gignac-Caille, A. M., & Oermann, M. H. (2001). Student and faculty perceptions of effective clinical instructors in ADN programs. *Journal of Nursing Education, 40,* 347–353.

Glendon, K., & Ulrich, D. (2004). Dear Florence: Tips and strategies for faculty. *Nurse Educator, 29,* 45–46.

Hamera, E., & Wright, T. (2004). Evaluation of the content and interaction in an online clinical conference for students in advanced psychiatric mental health nursing. *Archives of Psychiatric Nursing, 18,* 4–10.

Johnson, D. W., & Johnson, F. P. (2003). *Joining together: Group theory and group skills* (8th ed.). Boston: Pearson.

Manias, E., & Aitken, R. (2005). Clinical teachers in specialty practice settings: Perceptions of their role within postgraduate nursing programs. *Learning in Health and Social Care, 4,* 67–77.

Mertler, C. A. (2003). *Classroom assessment.* Los Angeles: Pyrczak.

O'Connor, A. B. (2006). *Clinical instruction and evaluation* (2nd ed.). Boston: Jones and Bartlett.

Oermann, M. H. (1997). Evaluating critical thinking in clinical practice. *Nurse Educator, 22,* 25–28.

Oermann, M. H. (2004). Using active learning in lecture: Best of "both worlds." *Journal of Nursing Education Scholarship, 1*(1), 1–11. Retrieved from http://www.bepress.com/ijnes/vol1/iss1/art1

Oermann, M. H., & Gaberson, K. (2006). *Evaluation and testing in nursing education* (2nd ed.). New York: Springer Publishing.

Oermann, M. H., Truesdell, S., & Ziolkowski, L. (2000). Strategy to assess, develop, and evaluate critical thinking. *Journal of Continuing Education in Nursing, 31,* 155–160.

Paul, R. W. (1993). *Critical thinking: How to prepare students for a rapidly changing world.* Santa Rosa, CA: Foundation for Critical Thinking.

Phillips, N., & Duke, M. (2001). The questioning skills of clinical teachers and preceptors: A comparative study. *Journal of Advanced Nursing, 33,* 523–529.

Profetto-McGrath, J., Smith, K. B., Day, R. A., & Yonge, O. (2004). The questioning skills of tutors and students in a context based baccalaureate nursing program. *Nurse Education Today, 24,* 363–372.

Rossignol, M. (2000). Verbal and cognitive activities between and among students and faculty in clinical conferences. *Journal of Nursing Education, 39,* 245–250.

Sellappah, S., Hussey, T., Blackmore, A. M., & McMurray, A. (1998). The use of questioning strategies by clinical teachers. *Journal of Advanced Nursing, 28,* 142–148.

Stiles, A. S. (2006). Cooperative learning: Enhancing individual learning through positive group process. In M. H. Oermann & K. T. Heinrich (Eds.), *Annual review of nursing education* (Vol. 4, pp. 131–159). New York: Springer Publishing.

Stokes, L., & Kost, G. (2005). Teaching in the clinical setting. In D. M. Billings & J. A. Halstead (Eds.), *Teaching in nursing: A guide for faculty* (2nd ed., pp. 325–346). St. Louis: Elsevier Saunders.

Wang, A. M., & Blumberg, P. (1983). A study on interaction techniques of nursing faculty in the clinical area. *Journal of Nursing Education, 22,* 144–150.

Ward, K. G., & Apsey, M. (2000). News, notes & tips. Fostering sensitivity in clinical conferencing. *Nurse Educator, 25,* 157, 169.

Wink, D. M. (1993). Using questioning as a teaching strategy. *Nurse Educator, 18,* 11–15.

Wink, D. M. (1995). The effective clinical conference. *Nursing Outlook, 43,* 29–32.

Wolff, A. (2007). Tutoring problem-based learning: A model for student-centered teaching. In L. E. Young & B. L. Paterson (Eds.), *Teaching nursing: Developing a student-centered learning environment* (pp. 242–278). Philadelphia: Lippincott Williams & Wilkins.

Chapter 13

Written Assignments

Written assignments enable students to learn about concepts and theories relevant to clinical practice, develop critical-thinking skills, and examine values and beliefs that may affect patient care. Written assignments about clinical practice combined with feedback from the teacher provide an effective means of developing students' writing abilities. While writing assignments may vary with each clinical course, depending on the outcomes of the course, assignments may be carefully sequenced across courses for students to develop their writing skills as they progress through the nursing program. The teacher is responsible for choosing written assignments that support the learning outcomes of the course and meet other curriculum goals.

PURPOSES OF WRITTEN ASSIGNMENTS

Written assignments for clinical learning have four main purposes: (1) assist students in understanding concepts and theories that relate to the care of their patients; (2) improve problem-solving and critical-thinking skills; (3) examine their own feelings, beliefs, and values generated from their clinical learning experiences; and (4) develop writing skills.

In choosing written assignments for clinical courses, the teacher should first consider the outcomes to be met through the assignments and the competencies that students need to develop in the course and nursing program. Writing assignments should build on one another to progressively develop students' skills. Another consideration is the number of assignments to be completed: How many assignments are needed to demonstrate mastery? It may be that one assignment well done is sufficient for meeting the outcomes of the clinical course, and students may then progress to other learning activities. Teachers should avoid using the same written assignments repeatedly throughout a clinical course and instead should choose assignments for specific learning outcomes.

Promote Understanding of Concepts and Theories

In written assignments students can describe concepts and theories relevant to the care of their patients and can explain how these concepts and theories guide their clinical decisions. Assignments for this purpose need a clear focus to prevent students merely summarizing and reporting what they read. Shorter assignments that direct students to apply particular concepts and theories to clinical practice may be of greater value in achieving this purpose than longer assignments for which students summarize readings they completed without any analysis of the meaning of those readings for their particular patients (Oermann, 2006). For instance, students may be asked to select an intervention for a patient with chronic pain and in one page provide a rationale for its use; read a research article related to care of one of their patients, critique the article, and report on their critique and why the research is or is not applicable to the patient's care; or select a family theory and complete an assessment of a family using this theory.

Improve Problem Solving and Critical Thinking

Written assignments provide an opportunity for students to analyze patient and other problems they have encountered in clinical practice, critique their interventions, and propose new approaches. In writing assignments, students may analyze data and clinical situations, identify additional assessment data needed for decision making, identify problems, propose alternate solutions, compare interventions, and evaluate the effectiveness of care. Writing assignments are particularly valuable for learning about evidence-based practice (EBP). Students can examine the evidence underlying different interventions and make decisions about the best approaches to use with their patients. Students can identify assumptions they made about patients' responses that influenced their clinical decisions, critique arguments, take a stand about an issue and develop a rationale to support it, and draw generalizations about patient care from different clinical experiences.

Assignments geared to critical thinking should give students freedom to develop their ideas and consider alternate perspectives. If the assignment is too restrictive, students are inhibited in their thinking and ways of approaching the problem.

Written assignments for critical thinking should be short, ranging from one to two paragraphs to a few pages. In developing these assignments, the teacher should avoid activities in which students merely report on the ideas of others. Instead, the assignment should ask students to consider an alternate point of view or a different way of approaching an issue. Short assignments also provide an opportunity for faculty to give prompt feedback to students on alternate ways of thinking about the clinical situation (Oermann, 2006).

In addition to being short, the assignment should focus on meeting a particular learning goal and should have specific directions to guide students' writing. For example, students may be asked to prepare a one-page paper comparing the physiological processes of asthma and bronchitis. Rather than writing on everything they read about asthma and bronchitis, students focus their papers on the physiology of these two conditions.

Examples of written assignments for problem solving and critical thinking follow:

- Compare data collected from two patients for whom you have recently cared. What are similarities and differences?

- Describe in one paragraph significant cues in the data you collected from your patient.

- Select one nursing diagnosis you identified for your patient and provide a rationale for it. What is one alternate diagnosis you might also consider and why? Complete this assignment in two typed pages.

- In one page, identify a patient for whom you have learned to provide care in this clinical course. Propose one alternate intervention and provide a rationale for its use.

- Compare, in no more than three pages, two interventions appropriate for your patient in terms of their rationale, research base, and effectiveness.

- Analyze an issue you faced in clinical practice, an alternate course of action that you could have used, and why this alternate action would also be effective (one-page paper).

- Identify an issue affecting your patient, family, or community. Analyze that issue from two different points of view. Provide a rationale for actions to be taken from both perspectives. How would you approach this issue and why?

- In no more than two paragraphs, list a decision you made today in your clinical practice and provide a rationale and evidence to support that decision.

Examine Feelings, Beliefs, and Values

Written assignments help learners examine feelings generated from caring for patients and reflect on their beliefs and values that might influence that care. Journals, for instance, provide a way for students to record their feelings about a patient or clinical activity and later reflect on these feelings. Assignments may be developed for students to identify their own beliefs and values and analyze how they affect their interactions with patients, families, and staff. Value-based statements may be given to students for written critique, or students may be asked to analyze an ethical issue, propose alternate courses of actions, and take a stand on the issue.

Develop Writing Skills

An important outcome of writing assignments is the development of skill in communicating ideas in written form. Assignments help students learn how to organize thoughts and present them clearly. This clarity in writing about clinical practice and care of patients develops through planned writing activities integrated in the nursing program. As a skill, writing ability requires practice, and students need to complete writing assignments across clinical courses. All too often, writing assignments are not sequenced progressively across courses or levels in the program; students, then, do not have the benefit of building writing skills sequentially.

Writing-to-learn programs are designed to meet the need for progressive development. In those programs, written assignments are sequenced across the nursing curriculum. Zygmont and Schaefer (2006) formulated a writing-across-the-curriculum project to develop students' critical-thinking and writing skills based on a model of critical thinking by Lynch and Wolcott (2001). In beginning nursing courses students complete writing assignments in which they define or list; for example, defining a problem in their words or listing facts related to a problem. As students progress through the program, the prompts for writing are at a higher cognitive level. Students might prepare a paper in which they synthesize information from the literature or explain the meaning of the data. Another useful strategy in Zygmont and Schaefer's writing program is the development of a writing portfolio where students keep all of their writing assignments, including corrected drafts and final graded papers.

A benefit of this planned approach to teaching writing is faculty feedback, provided through drafts and rewrites of papers. Drafts are essential to foster development of writing skill. Drafts should be critiqued by faculty for accuracy of content, development of ideas, organization, clarity of expression, and writing skills such as sentence structure, punctuation, and spelling (Oermann, 2002).

Small group critique of one another's writing is also appropriate particularly for formative purposes. This small group critique provides a basis for subsequent revisions and gives feedback to students about both content and writing style. While students may not identify every error in sentence structure and punctuation, they can provide valuable feedback on content, organization, how the ideas are developed, and clarity of writing. If the assignment will be graded at a later point, students may use the grading criteria as a guideline for their peer review.

TYPES OF WRITING ASSIGNMENTS FOR CLINICAL LEARNING

There are many types of writing assignments appropriate for enhancing clinical learning. Some of these assignments help students learn the content they are writing about but do not necessarily improve writing skill, and other assignments also promote competency in writing. For example, structured assignments such as care plans provide minimal opportunity for freedom of expression, originality, and creativity. Other assignments, though, such as term papers on clinical topics, promote understanding of new content and its use in clinical practice as well as writing ability.

Types of written assignments for clinical learning include concept map, concept analysis paper, short written assignments, nursing care plan, case method and study, evidence-based practice (EBP) papers, teaching plan, journal, group writing, and portfolio.

Concept Map

A *concept map* is a graphic or pictorial arrangement of key concepts related to a patient's care. By developing a concept map, students can visualize how signs and symptoms, problems, interventions, medications, and other aspects of a patient's care relate to one another. Concept maps help students organize patient information.

There are many uses of concept maps in clinical learning. First, students may complete a concept map from their readings to assist them in linking new facts and concepts to their own patients. The readings students complete for clinical practice, and in nursing courses overall, contain vast amounts of facts and specific information; concept maps help students process this information in a meaningful way, linking new and existing ideas together.

Second, concept maps are useful in helping students prepare for clinical prac-tice. All, Huycke, and Fisher (2003) suggest that the concept map be presented in preclinical conference, revised during the clinical learning activity, and then dis-cussed in postclinical conference.

Third, concept maps may be developed collaboratively by students in clini-cal conferences. For this purpose, students may present a patient for whom they have cared, with the clinical group then developing a concept map about that pa-tient's care. Or the clinical group may develop a concept map about conditions or community problems they are learning about in the course. As another strategy, students can present the concept maps they developed for their patients, and the group can analyze and discuss them. Critiquing each others' concept maps enhances critical thinking, learning from one another, and group process; it also allows for feedback from the teacher and peers.

Concept maps are organized with specific concepts written under more general ones. Students first identify relevant concepts for their patients' care and then link these concepts together. Different types of lines can be used to illus-trate the relationships among the concepts. Figure 13.1 shows a sample concept map.

Concept maps are most appropriately used for formative evaluation. How-ever, Couey (2004) suggested that students can write short papers about the inter-relationships among the concepts, which then could be graded by faculty.

Concept Analysis Paper

Concept analysis papers help students understand difficult concepts and how they are applied in patient care. For these papers, students identify and define a concept related to clinical practice, such as family-centered care or a diagnosis such as bron-chitis. They then explore characteristics of the concept and how that concept would be seen in clinical practice. Students can write papers about the concept and can develop case studies that exemplify its various characteristics. Students might relate a concept described in class or their readings to their own patients and pre-pare a paper on similarities and differences between what they learned and their patients. Here is an assignment example:

> Choose a concept from your textbook that is relevant to a patient you cared for in clinical practice last week. Write a one-page paper on how that con-cept relates to your patient. What were similarities and differences between the textbook description of the concept and what you found in caring for this patient?

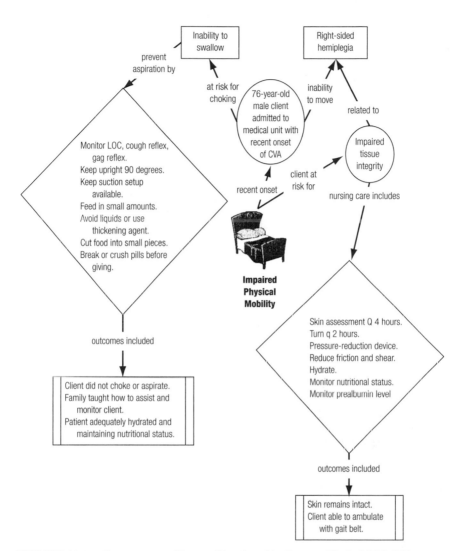

FIGURE 13.1   Concept map. (*Source:* Developed by Deanne Blach, MSN, RN. Reprinted with permission of Deanne Blach, 2006.)

Short Written Assignments

Short written assignments in clinical courses are valuable for promoting critical thinking and analysis. Short assignments avoid students summarizing what others have written without thinking about the content themselves (Oermann, 2006). With a short assignment, students can compare diagnoses, compare interventions with their evidence, explore decisions that might be made in a clinical situation, analyze an issue and approaches, and analyze a case scenario, among many other types. Sample assignments are found in Table 13.1.

Writing assignments can be critiqued by the teacher or by peers for formative evaluation. Students can often suggest other ways of viewing the clinical situation and can identify content or writing that is unclear. For grading purposes, though, short papers should be evaluated by the teacher.

TABLE 13.1   Examples of Short Written Assignments for Clinical Courses

List the interventions you used today for your patient. What evidence supports each of those interventions? Summarize the evidence and its strength. Identify one other intervention that would be appropriate and provide a rationale for its use. (1 page)

Select one concept or theory presented in your textbook or in class that helps you better understand your patient's problems. In no more than two paragraphs, explain how you would *use* that concept or theory in your patient's care.

Describe in one page how your patient's problems, treatments, and interventions are similar to or different from your readings and why.

In a clinical conference present (face-to-face or online) your assessment of one of your patients. [Other students in the clinical group write possible diagnoses, supporting data that were presented, and additional data needed to confirm their proposed diagnoses. Students pass the writing to a peer to critique and refine as needed.] Lead a discussion comparing students' diagnoses and supporting data with what was listed in the medical record, your own analysis, and your experience in caring for that patient.

Write a letter to the editor of journal about an article published in the most recent issue that addresses a clinical practice problem. Provide information about the issue from an additional published source not cited in the article, or from your own experience. Include the editor's name and journal title.

Develop a protocol for patient care based on your readings and class discussions. What evidence did you use to develop your protocol? Include your information sources. Bring the protocol to postclinical conference for critique by peers. (1 page)

TABLE 13.1   (Continued)

Sample Short Scenarios for Students to Respond to in Writing

You are the manager on a 24-bed medical-surgical unit, always in need of RN staff. In a one-page paper, explain how you would respond, using two different management theories, to staff nurse A in the following scenario: In a meeting at the beginning of the shift, staff nurse A comes to you and complains about having to work with two of the nursing assistants assigned to her team. She asks you to reassign those assistants to another team and requests two other assistants for that day.

Mr. S refuses to get out of bed to walk to the bathroom—he is in "too much pain." In report, however, the nurse indicated Mr. S walked himself to the bathroom twice during the night. What are three different ways of handling this situation? What are possible consequences of each? What would you do and why? (1/2 page)

You are helping one of the other nurses, who is a friend of yours, finish up his care so you can go to dinner together. You notice that your friend moves from patient to patient without washing his hands. When you tell him about this, he responds that none of his patients have any infections. What should you do? Why did you choose this approach? (2 paragraphs)

The unit policy is to restrict visitors at certain times of the day. Some of the nurses want to have open visiting hours. Develop a position paper that supports open visitation for families and a second one that argues against the recommendation. (maximum length 2 pages)

Source: From Oermann, M. H. (2006). Short written assignments for clinical nursing courses. *Nurse Educator, 31,* 228–231. Reprinted by permission of Lippincott Williams & Wilkins, 2006.

Nursing Care Plan

Nursing care plans enable students to analyze patients' health problems and design plans of care. With care plans students can record assessment data, identify relevant nursing diagnoses, select evidence-based interventions and consider how they interface with other disciplines, and identify outcomes to be measured. Care plans should be usable—they should guide students' planning of their patients' care, be realistic, and be able to be implemented in the health care setting.

Completing a written care plan may help the student identify nursing and other interventions for specific problems, but whether that same care plan promotes problem-solving learning and critical thinking is questionable. Often students develop their care plans from the literature or ones already completed in the clinical setting without thinking about the content themselves. Even if the care plan is the most appropriate written assignment for the course outcomes, the question remains as to how many care plans students need to complete in a clinical course to meet those learning goals. Once the goals have been achieved, then other written assignments may be more effective for clinical learning.

Case Method and Case Study

Case method and case study describe a clinical situation developed around an actual or a hypothetical patient for student review and critique. In case method, the case provided for analysis is generally shorter and more specific than in case study. Case studies are more comprehensive in nature, thereby presenting a complete picture of the patient and clinical situation. After analyzing the case, students complete written questions about it; questions may be answered individually or by small groups of students. Case method and case study are discussed in detail in Chapter 11.

Evidence-Based Practice Papers

Assignments in clinical courses can guide students' learning about EBP and its use in patient care. Studies continue to reveal the limited understanding of nurses about EBP and their reliance on colleagues for guidance with clinical decisions rather than on research and other sources of evidence (Estabrooks, Chong, Brigidear, & Profetto-McGrath, 2005; Pravikoff, Tanner, & Pierce, 2005). Clinical assignments that are integrated in courses throughout the nursing program foster students' knowledge about EBP and its importance in clinical practice.

A useful model for planning EBP assignments for clinical courses was developed by Pierce (2005). This model includes five steps, which Pierce suggests are critical to implementing EBP in a nursing curriculum:

1. Develop a researchable question about clinical practice.
2. Design and complete an evidence search.
3. Retrieve and evaluate the evidence.
4. Use the evidence for clinical decisions.
5. Evaluate effects of decision on patient outcomes.

Student assignments can be developed for each of these steps and integrated in clinical courses in the program. By using a model such as this one or another EBP model, teachers can plan assignments for each clinical course in the curriculum, assisting students in integrating EBP into their practice. Table 13.2 provides sample clinical assignments based on this model.

TABLE 13.2   Sample Clinical Assignments for Learning About Evidence-Based Practice

Develop a Researchable Question About Clinical Practice

Identify a problem of one of your patients. What additional information do you need to plan care, and why is this information critical to your decision making? How will you find this information?

Think about a patient you cared for this week. Identify a question you had about that patient's care. List two sources of information to answer that question with a rationale for why these sources are appropriate. Discuss your question, sources of information, and rationale with a peer during postclinical conference. Are there other sources of information? Present to the clinical group.

Identify a change in practice needed on your unit. Why is it needed? What led you to this decision? Write a short paper. (no more than 1 page)

Design and Complete an Evidence Search

List a question you had about a patient's care. Identify key words to search for an answer. Go to the Cumulative Index to Nursing and Allied Health Literature (CINAHL) and modify your key words as needed. Complete the search in CINAHL, mapping out your search strategy. Summarize your findings. What would you do differently with this search the next time? Write a two- to three-page paper on this search and what you found.

Conduct the same search in Medline. What are the differences, if any, in the results of your search? What did you learn about these two databases? Present in clinical conference.

Identify a bibliographic database other than CINAHL or Medline that you might use in your clinical practice, e.g., PsycINFO. Identify a question that could be answered by searching in that database. Conduct the search and summarize your results. How could you use these results in clinical practice? What did you learn about this database? Present in online discussion.

Retrieve and Evaluate the Evidence

Identify a question about clinical practice or a change in practice that might be indicated. Review the literature. What studies are relevant for inclusion in your review and why? Critique the evidence (consider validity, relevance, and applicability). Summarize your findings and develop a written proposal for use of this evidence to guide practice or why a practice change is not indicated.

Review clinical research studies in an area of nursing practice related to the course. Critically appraise those studies and synthesize findings. What are issues in implementing those findings in your clinical setting? What would you propose to facilitate implementation? Prepare a paper on your review and analysis.

(continues)

TABLE 13.2   Sample Clinical Assignments for Learning About Evidence-Based Practice (Continued)

Discuss how you might use the Cochrane Database of Systematic Reviews in your patient care. Select a nursing intervention and locate information about this intervention in Cochrane. Write a report on your findings. (3–4 pages)

Use the Evidence for Clinical Decisions

List interventions for one of your patients. What is the evidence base for *each* of these? Provide a rationale for their use based on the strength of the evidence. Include the sources of information you used to determine the evidence base. What evidence is missing, and what do you propose?

Review your patient's care. Select one problem not adequately met with current practices. Search for evidence to suggest a change in practice, evaluate the evidence, and write a paper about how you would change practice based on your review. What would you do differently next time you cared for that patient or patients with similar problems?

Select an intervention and find evidence using resources from the Joanna Briggs Institute. Describe the evidence you located. Did it help you make a decision about the effectiveness of the intervention? Why or why not? How would you use this information in your clinical practice? Prepare a short paper.

Evaluate Effects of Decisions on Patient Outcomes

For a practice change or evidence-based intervention you proposed in an earlier assignment, plan how you would evaluate its effect on patient outcomes. Present in online discussion.

Identify a question you had about your patient's care. Go to the National Guideline Clearinghouse. What evidence-based practice guidelines are relevant for this patient? If you implemented one of these guidelines in your clinical setting, what outcomes would you measure?

Implement one evidence-based intervention in patient care and evaluate its outcomes. Write a short report on your findings. (not more than 2 pages)

Source: Based on a model developed by Pierce, S. T. (2005). Integrating evidence-based practice into nursing curricula. In M. H. Oermann & K. T. Heinrich (Eds.), *Annual review of nursing education* (Vol. 3, pp. 233–248). New York: Springer Publishing.

Teaching Plan

Teaching plans, which may be completed individually or in small groups, enable students to apply concepts of learning and teaching to patients, families, and communities. After developing the teaching plan, students may use it as a basis for their teaching. There are many formats for teaching plans, but the assignment would typically include these parts: objectives, content, teaching strategies, and evaluation strategies.

Journal

Journal writing assists students in relating theory to clinical practice, linking their classroom and online instruction to care of patients, and in reflecting on their clinical learning activities. When students reexamine their clinical decisions and propose alternative actions, journaling also encourages the development of critical-thinking and problem-solving skills.

Writing in journals about clinical practice provides opportunities for students to

- document feelings generated from their clinical practice,

- describe perceptions of patients and clinical experiences,

- record accomplishments in clinical practice,

- develop values and affective skills,

- communicate with the clinical teacher.

Journals are also a good strategy for developing reflective practice (Blake, 2005; Kessler & Lund, 2004). In a journal, students can reflect back on their experiences and reexamine them, improving their awareness of own behaviors and responses within the context of the clinical environment. Through a reflective journal, students can

- find meaning in their clinical experiences,

- make connections between those experiences and their learning in the classroom,

- gain values of the nursing profession and develop their own affective skills;

- learn about the perspectives of others,

- reflect on the roles of the nurse as a professional,

- develop critical thinking skills,

- learn to care for themselves (Blake, 2006, p. 2).

Daroszewski, Kinser, and Lloyd (2004) used online journaling for sharing clinical experiences in an advanced practice nursing course, promoting discussions, and mentoring students, among other outcomes. Students kept a weekly online journal, which was on the course Web site discussion board. Each journal entry included specific objectives, clinical activities, students' reflection on those experiences, and discussion of them. The journals were open to other students in the course, who commented on at least two of their peers' journal entries. While there was only a small group of students ($N = 6$) who evaluated this method, they were positive about its value. One of the benefits was the opportunity to learn what other students were doing in their clinical practicum.

There are different ways of structuring journals, and the choice of structure should be based on the intended outcomes of using the journal in the clinical course. The first step for the teacher is to identify the learning outcomes to be met through journal writing, such as reflecting on clinical decisions or describing feelings in caring for a patient, and then how journal entries should be made. Students should understand what learning outcomes are being achieved through journaling so they can gear their entries to those goals.

Journals are typically not graded but provide an opportunity for giving feedback to learners and developing a dialogue with them. Students have greater freedom in recording feelings, ideas, and responses when the journal is used only for feedback. Faculty members are responsible for providing thoughtful and prompt feedback similar to any written assignment.

Group Writing

Not all writing assignments need to be done by students individually. There is much to be gained with group writing exercises as long as the groups are small and the exercises are carefully focused. Short written assignments, such as analyzing an issue and reporting in writing the outcomes of the analysis or developing a care plan or teaching protocol as a group, may be completed in clinical conferences. These group assignments provide opportunities for students to express their ideas to others in the group and work collaboratively to communicate the results of their thinking as a group in written form.

Portfolio

A portfolio provides an opportunity for students to present projects they completed in their clinical courses over a period of time. Portfolios may include evidence of student learning for a series of clinical learning activities over the duration of a clinical course or for documenting competencies in terms of curriculum or program outcomes (Oermann & Gaberson, 2006).

There are two types of portfolios: best-work and growth and learning progress (Nitko, 2004). Best-work portfolios include materials and products developed by students in clinical practice that demonstrate their learning and achievements. These portfolios reflect the best work of the students in the clinical course. In contrast, growth and learning-progress portfolios include materials and products in the process of being developed. These portfolios serve as a way of monitoring students' progress in clinical practice (Oermann & Gaberson, 2006). With both types of portfolios, the teacher reviews them periodically and provides feedback on the materials and products in the portfolio.

The content of the portfolio depends on the goals to be achieved. Students may include in their portfolios any materials they developed individually or in a group that provide evidence of their achieving the outcomes of the clinical course or demonstrating the clinical competencies. Examples of these materials are

- documents that students developed for patient care,

- teaching plans and materials,

- papers written about clinical practice,

- selected journal entries,

- reports of group work and products,

- reports and observations made in the clinical setting,

- a self-assessment,

- reflections of their patient care experiences and meaning to them,

- other products that demonstrate their clinical competencies and what they learned in the course.

Table 13.3 presents a process for developing a portfolio for a clinical course.

TABLE 13.3   Developing a Portfolio for Clinical Learning

Step 1: Identify the purposes of the portfolio.

- Will the portfolio serve as a means of monitoring students' development of clinical competencies, focusing predominantly on the growth of students? Will the portfolio provide evidence of students' best work in clinical practice, including products reflecting their learning over a period of time? Or will the portfolio meet both demands, enabling the teacher to give continual feedback to students on the process of learning and projects on which they are working as well as providing evidence of their accomplishments and achievements in clinical practice?
- Will the portfolio be used for formative or summative evaluation? Or both?
- Will the portfolio be developed for a series of clinical learning activities, over the length of a clinical course, or over the length of the curriculum?
- Will the portfolio serve as a means of assessing prior learning and therefore have an impact on the types of learning activities or courses that students complete, for instance, for assessing the prior learning of RNs entering a baccalaureate or higher degree program or for licensed practical nurses entering an associate degree program?
- What is the student's role in defining the focus and content of the portfolio?

Step 2: Identify the types of entries and content to be included in the portfolio.

- What types of entries are required in the portfolio, for example, products developed by students, descriptions of projects with which students are involved, descriptions of clinical learning activities and reactions to them, observations made in clinical practice and analysis of them, and papers completed by students?
- In addition to required entries, what other types of content and entries might be included in the portfolio?
- Who determines the content of the portfolio and types of entries? Teacher only? Student only? Both?
- Will the entries be the same for all students or individualized by the student?
- What is the minimum number of entries?
- How should the entries in the portfolio be organized, or will students organize it themselves?
- What is the time frame for each entry to be included in the portfolio and at what points in time should it be submitted to faculty for review and feedback?
- Will teacher and student meet in a conference for discussion of the portfolio?

Step 3: Decide on the evaluation of the portfolio entries, including criteria for evaluation of individual entries and the portfolio overall.

- How will the portfolio be integrated within the clinical evaluation grade and course grade, if at all?
- What criteria will be used to evaluate, and perhaps score, each type of entry and the portfolio as a whole?
- Will only the teacher evaluate the portfolio and its entries? Or will students evaluate their own progress and work? Or will the evaluation be a collaborative effort?

Source: Adapted from Oermann, M. H., & Gaberson, K. B. (2006). *Evaluation and testing in nursing education* (2nd ed., pp. 235–236). New York: Springer Publishing. Adapted by permission of Springer Publishing Company, Inc., New York.

EVALUATING WRITTEN ASSIGNMENTS

Written assignments may be evaluated formatively or summatively. Formative evaluation provides feedback to students for their continued learning but not for grading purposes. Periodic assessment of drafts of papers and work in progress is formative in nature and is not intended for arriving at a grade. Summative evaluation of completed writing assignments is designed for grading the assignment, not for giving feedback to the student.

For written assignments that are not graded, the teacher's role is to give prompt and sufficient feedback for students to learn from the assignment. If the assignment will be graded at a later time, however, then criteria for grading should be established and communicated to the learner. Any assignment that will eventually be graded should have clear, specific, and measurable criteria for evaluation. Some writing assignments, such as journals, do not lend themselves to grading and instead are best used for formative evaluation only.

Drafts

If drafts of written assignments are to be submitted, the teacher should inform students of each required due date. All written assignments benefit from prompt and specific feedback from the teacher. Feedback should be given on the quality of the content, as reflected in the criteria for evaluation, and on writing style if appropriate for the assignment. Students need specific suggestions about revisions, not general statements such as "Unclear objectives in teaching plan." Instead, tell students exactly what needs to be changed, for instance, "Objective #1 in teaching plan is not measurable. Revise the verb; content is clear and relevant." Drafts of written assignments are important because they serve as a means of improving writing and thinking about the content. Prompt, clear, and specific feedback about revisions is essential to meet this purpose. Drafts in most instances are used for feedback and therefore are not graded.

Criteria for Evaluation

The criteria for evaluation should relate to the learning outcomes to be met with the assignment. For example, if students write a short paper to meet the objective, "Compare interventions for nausea associated with chemotherapy," criteria should relate to the appropriateness and evidence base of the interventions selected for critique, how effectively the student compared them, the rationale developed for the analysis, and the like.

General criteria for evaluating written assignments follow. These criteria need to be adapted based on the type of assignment and its intent. For assignments that are graded, students should have the criteria for evaluation and scoring protocol or rubric at the time the assignment is made so they can develop it with these criteria in mind.

1. *Content*

    Content is relevant.

    Content is accurate.

    Significant concepts and theories are presented.

    Concepts and theories are applied to clinical situation and used for the analysis.

    Content is comprehensive.

    Content reflects current research.

    Hypotheses, conclusions, and decisions are supported.

    Content is individualized to patient, family, or community

2. *Organization*

    Content is organized logically.

    Ideas are presented in a logical sequence.

    Ideas are described clearly.

3. *Process*

    Process used to arrive at solutions, approaches, decisions, and so forth is adequate.

    Consequences of decisions are considered and weighed.

    A sound rationale is provided.

    For papers on analysis of issues, the rationale supports the position taken.

    Multiple perspectives and new approaches are considered.

4. *Writing Style*

    Sentence structure is clear.

    There are no grammatical errors.

    There are no spelling errors.

    Appropriate punctuation is used.

    The length of the paper is consistent with requirements.

    References are cited appropriately throughout the paper.

    References are cited accurately according to the required format.

Grading Assignments

In grading written assignments, a scoring protocol should be developed based on the criteria established for evaluation. The protocol should include the elements to be evaluated and points allotted for each one. The scoring protocol must be used in the same way for all students. This is an important principle in grading written assignments to assure consistency across papers and to focus the evaluation on the specific criteria. Some teachers tend to be more lenient, and others tend to be more critical in their review of papers. A scoring protocol helps the teacher base the grade on the established criteria rather than on some other standard. Teachers will be more consistent in grading papers if they first establish specific criteria for evaluation, then develop a scoring protocol based on these criteria, and, lastly, use that scoring protocol in the same way for each student.

For some papers a scoring rubric might be developed to guide the evaluation. A *rubric* is a scoring guide for evaluating a paper and other types of performance (Mertler, 2003). With a holistic rubric the teacher scores the paper as a whole without assessing individual parts and elements of the paper. An analytic rubric guides the assessment of separate parts of the paper and then sums them for a total score (Mertler). For short written assignments in clinical courses, a protocol for scoring them is sufficient. However, for term papers or longer written assignments, the teacher can develop a more detailed rubric for use in evaluating them.

Written assignments that are graded should be read anonymously if at all possible, but anonymity is sometimes difficult to achieve with small groups of students. Nevertheless, students can record their student numbers on their papers rather than their names. There is a tendency in evaluating papers and other written assignments, similar to essay items, for the teacher to be influenced by a general impression of the student. This is called the halo effect. The teacher may have positive or negative feelings about the student or other biases that may influence evaluating and grading the assignment.

Another reason to read papers anonymously is to avoid a carryover effect. In this situation the teacher carries an impression of the quality of one written assignment to the next one that the student completes. If the student develops an outstanding paper, the teacher may be influenced to score subsequent written assignments at a similarly high level; the same situation may occur with a poor paper. The teacher therefore carries the impression of the student from one written assignment to the next. If there are multiple questions that students answered as part of a written assignment, the previous scores should be covered to avoid being biased about the quality of the next answer. In addition the teacher should evaluate all students' answers to one question before proceeding to the next question (Oermann & Gaberson, 2006).

All written assignments should be read twice before scoring. In the first reading, it is important to note errors in content, omission of major content areas, problems with organization, problems with the process used for approaching the problem or issue, and problems with writing style. Comments can be recorded on the student's paper with suggestions for revision. After reading through all of the papers, then the teacher should begin a second reading for scoring purposes.

Papers and other types of written assignments should be read in random order. After the first reading, the teacher can shuffle the papers so they are read in a random order the second time through. Papers read early may be scored higher than those read near the end (Oermann & Gaberson, 2006). Teacher fatigue also may set in and influence grading of the papers. While this section of the chapter deals with grading written assignments, the teacher should remember that many of these assignments will not be graded.

SUMMARY

Written assignments for clinical learning have four main purposes: to learn about concepts and theories relevant to clinical practice, develop critical-thinking skills, examine values and beliefs that may affect patient care, and, with some assignments, develop writing skills. Not all writing assignments achieve each of these outcomes. The teacher decides first on the outcomes to be met, then plans the writing assignment with these outcomes in mind.

Written assignments for critical thinking should be short. In developing these assignments, the teacher should avoid activities in which students merely report on the ideas of others; instead, the assignment should ask students to consider an alternate point of view or a different way of approaching an issue. Short assignments also provide an opportunity for faculty to give prompt feedback to students.

Written assignments help learners examine feelings generated from caring for patients and reflect on their beliefs and values that might influence that care. They also help students learn how to organize thoughts and present them clearly. Some faculty members have developed writing-to-learn programs in which written assignments are sequenced across the nursing curriculum.

There are many types of written assignments that can be used for clinical learning. Concept map, concept analysis paper, short written assignments, nursing care plan, case method and study, EBP practice papers, teaching plan, journal, group writing, and portfolio were presented in this chapter.

Written assignments may be evaluated formatively or summatively. Formative evaluation provides feedback to students for their continued learning but not for grading purposes. Periodic assessment of drafts of papers and work in progress is formative in nature and is not intended for arriving at a grade. Summative evaluation of completed writing assignments is designed for grading the assignment, not for giving feedback to the student.

In grading written assignments, a scoring protocol should be developed based on the criteria established for evaluation. The scoring protocol must be used in the same way for all students. Many written assignments, though, are not graded.

REFERENCES

All, A. C., Huycke, L. I., & Fisher, M. J. (2003). Instructional tools for nursing education: Concept maps. *Nursing Education Perspectives, 24,* 311–317.

Blake, T. K. (2005). Journaling: An active learning technique. *International Journal of Nursing Education Scholarship, 2*(1), Article 7.

Couey, D. (2004). Using concept maps to foster critical thinking. In L. Caputi & L. Engelmann (Eds.), *Teaching nursing: The art and science* (pp. 634–651). Glen Ellyn, IL: College of DuPage Press.

Daroszewski, E. B., Kinser, A. G., & Lloyd, S. L. (2004). Online, directed journaling in community health advanced practice nursing clinical education. *Journal of Nursing Education, 43,* 175–180.

Estabrooks, C. A., Chong, H., Brigidear, K. & Profetto-McGrath, J. (2005). Profiling Canadian nurses' preferred knowledge sources for clinical practice. *Canadian Journal of Nursing Research, 37,* 118–140.

Kessler, P. D., & Lund, C. H. (2004). Reflective journaling: Developing an online journal for distance education. *Nurse Educator, 29,* 20–24.

Lynch, C. L., & Wolcott, S. K. (2001, October). *Helping your students develop critical thinking skills. Idea Paper #37.* Manhattan, KS: The IDEA Center.

Mertler, C. A. (2003). *Classroom assessment: A practical guide for educators.* Los Angeles: Pyrczak.

Nitko, A. J. (2004). *Educational assessment of students* (4th ed.). Upper Saddle River, NJ: Prentice Hall.

Oermann, M. H. (2002). *Writing for publication in nursing.* Philadelphia: Lippincott, Williams & Wilkins.

Oermann, M. H. (2004). Using active learning in lecture: Best of "both worlds." *Journal of Nursing Education Scholarship, 1*(1), 1–11. Retrieved from http://www.bepress.com/ijnes/vol1/iss1/art1

Oermann, M. H. (2006). Short written assignments for clinical nursing courses. *Nurse Educator, 31,* 228–231.

Oermann, M. H., & Gaberson, K. B. (2006). *Evaluation and testing in nursing education* (2nd ed.). New York: Springer Publishing.

Pierce, S. T. (2005). Integrating evidence-based practice into nursing curricula. In M. H. Oermann & K. T. Heinrich (Eds.), *Annual review of nursing education* (Vol. 3, pp. 233–248). New York: Springer Publishing.

Pravikoff, D. S., Tanner, A. B., & Pierce, S. T. (2005). Readiness of U.S. nurses for evidence-based practice. *American Journal of Nursing, 105*, 40–51.

Zygmont, D. M., & Schaefer, K. M. (2006). Writing across the nursing curriculum project. In M. H. Oermann & K. T. Heinrich (Eds.), *Annual review of nursing education* (Vol. 4, pp. 275–290). New York: Springer Publishing.

Chapter 14

Using Preceptors in Clinical Teaching

As discussed in Chapter 4, the preceptor teaching model is an alternative to the traditional clinical teaching model. It is based on the assumption that a consistent one-to-one relationship between an experienced nurse and a nursing student or novice staff nurse is an effective method of providing individualized guidance in clinical learning as well as opportunities for professional socialization (Kersbergen & Hrobsky, 1996; Stokes & Kost, 2004). Preceptorships have been used extensively with senior nursing students, graduate students preparing for advanced practice roles, and new staff nurse orientees, but they have also been used effectively with beginning nursing students (Kersbergen & Hrobsky, 1996; LeGris & Côte, 1997; Nordgren, Richardson, & Laurella, 1998; Stokes & Kost, 2004). This chapter discusses the effective use of preceptors as clinical teachers. The advantages and disadvantages of preceptorships are examined, and suggestions are made for selecting, preparing, evaluating, and rewarding preceptors.

PRECEPTORSHIP MODEL OF CLINICAL TEACHING

A *preceptorship* is a time-limited, one-to-one relationship between a learner and an experienced nurse who is employed by the health care agency in which the learning activities take place. The teacher is not physically present during the clinical learning activities; the preceptor provides intensive, individualized learning opportunities that improve the learner's clinical competence and confidence. Regardless of learners' levels of education and experience, preceptorships provide opportunities for socialization into professional nursing roles (LeGris & Côte, 1997; Nordgren, et al., 1998; Stokes & Kost, 2004).

In a preceptorship model, the teacher is a faculty member or educator who has overall responsibility for the quality of the clinical teaching and learning. The teacher provides the link between the educational program and the practice setting by selecting and preparing preceptors, assigning students to preceptors, providing guidance for the selection of appropriate learning activities, serving as a resource to the preceptor–student pair, and evaluating student and preceptor performance. The preceptor functions as a role model and provides individualized clinical instruction, support, and socialization for the learner (Stokes & Kost, 2004). The preceptor also participates in evaluation of learner performance, although the teacher has ultimate responsibility for summative evaluation decisions.

In academic programs that prepare nurses for initial entry into practice, preceptorships are generally used for students in their last semester, but providing preceptors for beginning students may have even greater benefits. Beginning students may gain from the individual attention of the preceptor and from assignments that help them to expand their basic skills, develop independence, and improve their self-confidence (Nordgren, Richardson, & Laurella, 1998). When preceptors effectively model such competencies as prioritization, they can help nursing students to develop their critical-thinking abilities (Myrick & Yonge, 2002).

Preceptorships are frequently used in graduate programs that prepare nurses for advanced clinical practice, administration, and education roles. At this level, a preceptorship involves well-defined learning objectives based on the student's past clinical, administrative, and teaching experience. The student observes and participates in learning activities that demonstrate functional role components, allowing rehearsal of role behaviors before actually assuming an advanced practice, administrative, or teaching role. The preceptor must be an expert practitioner who can model the role functions of advanced practice nurses, including decision making, leadership, teaching, problem solving, and scholarship.

In many health care organizations, preceptors participate in the orientation of newly hired staff nurses. Preceptors in these settings act as role models for new staff nurses and support them in their transition into professional practice or socialization into new roles. Preceptors work one-to-one with new staff nurses, but there is wide variation in the scope of the preceptor role. In some settings, the preceptor is merely a more experienced peer who works side by side with the orientee; in other settings, the preceptor role is more formally that of clinical teacher. Successful preceptorship programs for new staff nurses can improve staff retention and recruitment (Bain, 1996; Hardy & Smith, 2001).

There are varied research findings on the effectiveness of the preceptor teaching model. Generally, studies indicate positive outcomes of students and new staff working with preceptors. Some early studies showed no difference in student performance between students assigned to preceptors and those taught in a traditional clinical teaching model. Some investigators presented anecdotal evidence from preceptors, teachers, and students that preceptorships enhanced student performance. Students who are assigned to preceptors usually report satisfaction due to increased confidence and independence (Stokes & Kost, 2004). However, students may also experience communication and interpersonal problems with their preceptors, and if these conflicts are not resolved successfully, negative outcomes can result (Mamchur & Myrick, 2003). The decision to use preceptors for clinical teaching should be based on the perceived benefits to students and the educational program, after a careful evaluation of the potential advantages and disadvantages.

ADVANTAGES AND DISADVANTAGES OF USING PRECEPTORS

The use of preceptors in clinical teaching has both advantages and disadvantages for the involved parties. Effective collaboration is required to minimize the drawbacks and achieve advantages for the preceptors, clinical agencies, students, and the educational program (LeGris & Côte, 1997).

Advantages and Disadvantages for Preceptors and Clinical Agencies

Preceptorships hold many potential advantages for preceptors and the clinical agencies that employ them. The presence of students in the clinical environment tends to enhance the professional development, leadership, and teaching skills of preceptors. While preceptors enjoy sharing their clinical knowledge and skill, they also appreciate the stimulation of working with students who challenge the status quo and raise questions about clinical practice. The interest and enthusiasm of students is often rewarding to nurses who take on the additional responsibilities of the preceptor role (LeGris & Côte, 1997). Students may assist preceptors with research or teaching projects. In agencies that use a clinical ladder, serving as a preceptor may be a means of advancing professionally within the system. The preceptorship model also produces opportunities to recruit potential staff members for the agency from among students who work with preceptors. Preceptorship programs for new staff nurses also produce positive outcomes. One hospital found that a structured preceptor program for new staff nurses in a medical intensive care unit improved the quality of care by promoting the professional development of both preceptors and preceptees (Hardy & Smith, 2001).

The greatest drawback of preceptorships to agencies and preceptors is usually the expected time commitment. Some clinical agencies may not agree to provide preceptors because of increased patient acuity and decreased staff levels, or potential preceptors may decline to participate because of the perception that to do so would add to their workloads (LeGris & Côte, 1997; Nordgren, et al., 1998).

Advantages and Disadvantages for Students

Students who participate in preceptorships enjoy a number of benefits. They have the advantage of working one-on-one with experts who can coach them to increased clinical competence and performance. Preceptorships also provide opportunities for students to experience the realities of clinical practice, including scheduling learning activities on evening and night shifts and weekends in order to follow their preceptors' schedules (LeGris & Côte, 1997; Nordgren, et al., 1998).

However, following their preceptors' schedules often creates conflicts with students' academic, work, and family commitments. Additionally, a preceptor's patient assignment may not be always appropriate for a student's clinical learning objectives (Nordgren, et al., 1998).

Advantages and Disadvantages for the Educational Program

Preceptorships offer many advantages for the educational program in which they are used. The use of preceptors provides more clinical teachers for students and thus more intensive guidance of students' learning activities. Working collaboratively with preceptors also helps faculty members to stay informed about the current realities of practice; up-to-date clinical information benefits ongoing curriculum development (LeGris & Côte, 1997).

Several disadvantages related to the use of preceptors may affect educational programs. Contrary to a common belief, teachers' responsibilities do not decrease when students work with preceptors. Initial selection of preceptors, preparation of preceptors and students, and ongoing collaboration and communication with preceptors and students require as much time as with the traditional clinical teaching model, or more. The preceptorship model requires considerable indirect teaching time for the development of relationships with agencies and preceptors and the evaluation of preceptors and students. When preceptors are used as clinical teachers, faculty members may be responsible for greater numbers of students in several clinical agencies and feel uncertain as to whether students are learning the application of theory and research findings to practice (LeGris & Côte, 1997; Nordgren, et al., 1998).

SELECTING PRECEPTORS

The success of preceptorships largely depends on the selection of appropriate preceptors; such selection is one of the teacher's most important responsibilities. Most faculty members consider the educational preparation of the preceptor to be important; most academic programs require the preceptor to have at least the degree for which the student is preparing, although insistence on this level of educational preparation does not guarantee that learners will be exposed only to professional role models.

The desire to teach and willingness to serve as a preceptor are important qualities of potential preceptors. Nurses who feel obligated to enact this role usually do not make enthusiastic, effective preceptors. Additional attributes of effective preceptors include the following (Bain, 1996; Stokes & Kost, 2004):

- *Clinical expertise or proficiency, depending on the level of the learner.* Preceptors should be able to demonstrate expert psychomotor, problem-solving, critical-thinking, and decision-making skills in their clinical practice. Nursing students and new staff nurses need preceptors who are at least proficient clinicians; graduate students need preceptors who are expert clinicians, administrators, or educators, depending on the goals of the preceptorship.
- *Leadership abilities.* Good preceptors are change agents in the health care organizations in which they are employed. They demonstrate effective communication skills and are trusted and respected by their peers.
- *Teaching skill.* Preceptors must understand and use principles of adult learning. They should be able to communicate ideas effectively to learners and give descriptive positive and negative feedback.
- *Professional role behaviors and attitudes.* Because preceptors act as role models for learners, they must demonstrate behaviors that represent important professional values. They are accountable for their actions and accept responsibility for their decisions. Good preceptors demonstrate maturity and self-confidence; their approach to learners is nonthreatening and nonjudgmental. Flexibility, open-mindedness, and a sense of humor are additional attributes of effective preceptors.

The selection of preceptor and setting should also take into account the learner's interest in a specific clinical specialty as well as the need for development of particular skills. The teacher may collaborate with nurse managers to select appropriate preceptors (Myrick & Yonge, 2003). It is wise not to choose preceptors from newly established units or those with recent high staff turnover.

PREPARING THE PARTICIPANTS

Thorough preparation of preceptors and students for their roles is another key to the success of preceptorships. Teachers are responsible for initial orientation and continuing support of all participants; preparation can be formal or informal.

Preceptors

Preparation of preceptors may begin with a general orientation, possibly for groups of potential preceptors at the selected agency. This orientation may include the following information:

- Benefits and challenges of precepting,

- Characteristics of a good preceptor,

- Principles of adult learning,

- Clinical teaching and evaluation methods,

- The preceptor's role in developing and implementing an individualized learning contract,

- The academic program curriculum structure, framework, and goals (LeGris & Côte, 1997; Stokes & Kost, 2004)

After preceptors have been selected, they need a specific orientation to their responsibilities. This orientation may take the form of a face-to-face or telephone conference with the teacher; written guidelines may be used to supplement the conference. Table 14.1 is an example of written guidelines for preceptors of graduate

TABLE 14.1   Sample Guidelines for a Preceptor of a Graduate Nursing Student

---

Guidelines for Preceptors—MSN Student Role Practicum

The preceptor is expected to do the following:
- Facilitate the student's entry into the health care organization.
- Provide the student with an orientation to the organization.
- After receiving the student's goals for the practicum, provide suggestions for how these goals can be accomplished.
- Assist the student with identifying a project that is consistent with organizational needs and student's interests, abilities, and learning needs.
- Meet with the student at regular intervals to discuss project progress and achievement of individual and course objectives.
- Provide the student with regular feedback regarding his or her performance.
- Communicate regularly with the faculty member regarding the student's progress.
- At the end of the preceptorship, provide a written evaluation of the student's performance related to goal achievement, clinical knowledge and skill, problem-solving and decision-making skills, communication and presentation skills, and interpersonal skills.

---

nursing students. The conference and written guidelines may include information such as the following:

- *The educational level and previous experience of the student.* Graduate students need learning activities that build on their previous learning and experience in order to produce advanced practice outcomes. Beginning students may not have developed the knowledge and skill to participate in all of the preceptor's activities. Nurses who have served as preceptors for new staff nurses may have expectations for nursing student performance that are unrealistically high (Case & Oermann, 2004).
- *How to choose specific learning activities based on learning objectives.* The teacher may share samples of learning contracts or lists of learning activities to guide the preceptor's selection of appropriate activities for the student. Kersbergen and Hrobsky (1996) proposed the use of a clinical map guide to planning precepted learning activities. Similar to critical pathways used by case managers in a managed care delivery system, clinical maps are tools that guide preceptors and students to select learning activities that meet identified objectives.
- *Scheduling of clinical learning activities.* A common feature of preceptorships is the scheduling of the student's learning activities according to the preceptor's work schedule. Preceptors should be advised of dates on which students and teachers may not be available because of school holidays, examinations, and other course requirements (Kersbergen & Hrobsky, 1996; LeGris & Côte, 1997; Nordgren, et al., 1998).

New preceptors have learning needs much like those of students and new staff nurses; supportive role models and coaching are essential to success. In fact, the teacher needs to "precept the preceptor" (Mamchur & Myrick, 2003, p. 194). Preceptor programs for newly hired staff nurses may hold regular meetings of preceptors with staff development instructors and nurse managers to review material such as adult learning principles, teaching and evaluation strategies, and conflict resolution.

Students

Learners also need to understand the purposes and process of the preceptorship. They need an orientation to the process of planning individual learning activities, an explanation of teacher and preceptor roles, and a review of unit policies specific to student practice (LeGris & Côte, 1997). At the beginning of the preceptorship, teachers should clarify evaluation responsibilities and expectations such as dates for learning contract approval, site visits, and conferences with faculty members.

IMPLEMENTATION

Successful implementation of preceptorships depends on mutual understanding of the roles and responsibilities of the participants. Teacher, student, and preceptor collaborate to plan and implement learning activities that will facilitate the student's goal attainment. Key to these processes is effective communication among the participants.

Roles and Responsibilities of Participants

Preceptors are responsible for patient care in addition to clinical teaching of the student. The preceptor is expected to be a positive role model and a resource person for the student. The clinical teaching responsibilities of the preceptor include creating a positive learning climate, including the student in activities that relate to learning goals, and providing feedback to the student and teacher. Sometimes preceptors experience conflict between the educator and evaluator roles, especially when precepting new staff members. If the learner is unable to perform according to expectations, the faculty member or staff development instructor must be notified so that a plan for correcting the deficiencies may be established (LeGris & Côte, 1997). In one study, preceptors were found to experience conflict in the preceptor–student relationship when they perceived a lack of competency on the part of the learner, related to the learner's knowledge and skill level (Mamchur & Myrick, 2003).

The student is expected to participate actively in planning learning activities. Planning may take the form of a learning contract that specifies individualized objectives and clinical learning activities. Because the teacher is not always present during learning activities, the student must communicate frequently with the teacher; communication may take the form of a reflective journal that is shared with teacher on a regular basis. The student must notify the teacher immediately of any problems encountered in the implementation of the preceptorship. In one study of conflict in preceptorships, Mamchur and Myrick (2003) found that 20% of students experienced conflict in their preceptorships but did not acknowledge or report it. In fact, preceptorship has been found to be among the most stressful of nursing student experiences (Yonge, Myrick, & Haase, 2002). According to Mamchur and Myrick (2003), students may not report conflict for several reasons:

- They perceive that they are expected to fit in to the practice setting with minimal disruption.

- They feel powerless and dependent on the preceptor's evaluation to complete the clinical practicum successfully.

- They fear receiving an unfavorable reference from the preceptor for future employment in that clinical agency.

The student's responsibilities also include self-evaluation and evaluation of the preceptor's teaching effectiveness, as is discussed later in this chapter.

As previously discussed, the teacher is responsible for making preceptor selections, pairing students with preceptors, and orienting preceptors and students. The teacher is an important resource to preceptors and students to assist in problem solving. The teacher must be alert to any sign of conflict in the student–preceptor relationship and promptly take a proactive role in resolving it. If a conflict cannot be resolved to the satisfaction of student, preceptor, and faculty member, the student's well-being should take precedence and, if necessary, the student should be reassigned (Mamchur & Myrick, 2003).

Teacher availability is particularly important if a problem arises at the clinical site that the preceptor and student cannot resolve. Therefore, the teacher must make arrangements for consultation via telephone, e-mail, or pager. The teacher also arranges individual and group conferences with students and preceptors, and visits the clinical sites as needed or requested by any of the participants. If students submit reflective journal entries, the teacher responds to them with feedback that helps students to evaluate their progress. Teachers have responsibility for the final evaluation of learner performance with input from preceptors, and they also evaluate the effectiveness of preceptors with input from students.

Planning and Implementing Learning Activities

A common strategy for planning and implementing students' learning activities in the preceptorship model of clinical teaching is the use of an individualized learning contract. A learning contract is an explicit agreement between teacher and student that clarifies expectations of each participant in the teaching–learning process. It specifies the learning goals that have been established, the learning activities selected to meet the objectives, and the expected outcomes and criteria by which they will be evaluated. In a preceptorship, the learning contract is negotiated among teacher, student, and preceptor, and serves as a guide for planning and implementing the student's learning activities. Table 14.2 is an example of a learning contract format that could be adapted for any level of learner.

As previously discussed, effective communication among the preceptor, student, and teacher is critical to the success of the preceptorship. Communication

TABLE 14.2   Sample Learning Contract Format

Learning Contract

Student Information
Name and credentials:

Address:

Phone number:

Fax number:

Email address:

Teacher Information
Name and credentials:

Address:

Phone number:

Fax number:

Email address:

Preceptor Information
Name and credentials:

Address:

Phone number:

Fax number:

Email address:

TABLE 14.2   (Continued)

Clinical Learning Objectives	Learning Activities and Resources	Evaluation Evidence, Responsibility, and Time Frame

Starting date:_____   Completion date: _____

Student Signature _____   Date_____

Preceptor Signature _____   Date_____

Teacher Signature _____   Date_____

between teacher and student may be facilitated by the student's keeping a reflective journal and sharing it with the teacher on a regular basis. In the journal, the student describes and analyzes learning activities that relate to the objective, reflecting on the meaning and value of the experiences. The journal entries may be recorded in a computer file, on paper or audiotape, or posted to an online discussion board; the teacher responds using the same media. Additionally, the student and teacher have telephone, e-mail, or face-to-face contact as necessary for the teacher to give consultation and guidance. Similarly, the teacher and preceptor should have regular contact by telephone, e-mail, or face-to-face meetings so that the teacher receives feedback about learner performance and offers guidance and consultation as needed.

The realities of clinical and academic cultures present challenges to effective communication among teacher, preceptor, and student. Preceptors often work a variety of shifts, students often have complicated academic and work schedules, and teachers have multiple responsibilities in addition to clinical teaching. Flexibility and commitment to establishing and maintaining communication are essential to overcome these challenges (LeGris & Côte, 1997).

EVALUATING THE OUTCOMES

Students, teachers, and preceptors share responsibility for monitoring the progress of learning and for evaluating outcomes of the preceptorship (LeGris & Côte, 1997). Student performance may be evaluated according to the terms specified in the learning contract or through the clinical evaluation methods used by the educational program. If a learning contract is used, student self-evaluation is usually an important strategy for assessing outcomes. As discussed earlier, preceptors are expected to give feedback to the learner and to the teacher, but the teacher has the responsibility for the summative evaluation of learner performance.

An important aspect of evaluation concerns the teaching effectiveness of preceptors. Students are an important source of information about the quality of their preceptors' clinical teaching, but the teacher should also assess the degree to which preceptors were able to effectively guide the students' learning. A modified form of the teaching effectiveness tool used to evaluate clinical teachers may be used to collect data from students regarding their preceptors (Nordgren, et al., 1998). Table 14.3 is an example of a form for student evaluation of preceptor teaching effectiveness. Because each preceptor typically is assigned to only one student at a time, it is usually impossible to maintain anonymity of student evaluations. Therefore, teachers may wish to share a summary of the student's evaluation, instead of the raw data, with the preceptor.

TABLE 14.3   Sample Tool for Student Evaluation of Preceptor Teaching Effectiveness

Student Evaluation of Preceptor's Teaching Effectiveness

Directions: Rate the extent to which each statement describes your preceptor's teaching behaviors by circling a number following each item, using the following scale:

4 = To a large extent
3 = To a moderate extent
2 = To a small extent
1 = Not at all

1. The preceptor was an excellent professional role model.	4 3 2 1
2. The preceptor guided my clinical problem solving.	4 3 2 1
3. The preceptor helped me to apply theory to clinical practice.	4 3 2 1
4. The preceptor was responsive to my individual learning needs.	4 3 2 1
5. The preceptor provided constructive feedback about my performance.	4 3 2 1
6. The preceptor communicated clearly and effectively.	4 3 2 1
7. The preceptor encouraged my independence.	4 3 2 1
8. The preceptor was flexible and open-minded.	4 3 2 1
9. Overall, the preceptor was an excellent clinical teacher.	4 3 2 1
10. I would recommend this preceptor for other students.	4 3 2 1

REWARDING PRECEPTORS

Preceptors make valuable contributions to nursing education programs, and they should receive appropriate rewards and incentives for their participation. At minimum, every preceptor should receive an individualized thank-you letter, specifying some of the benefits that the student received from the preceptorship. A copy of the letter may be sent to the preceptor's supervisor or manager to be used as evidence of clinical excellence at the time of the preceptor's next performance evaluation.

Other formal and informal ways of acknowledging the contributions of preceptors for nursing students and new staff members include

- a name badge that identifies the nurse as a preceptor;

- a certificate of appreciation, signed by the administrator of the nursing education program or the staff development program;

- an annual preceptor recognition event, including refreshments and an inspirational speaker;

- free or reduced-price registration for continuing education programs offered by the nursing education program or clinical facility;

- travel expenses and registration fees to attend professional development conferences off-site;

- educational leave time for academic and continuing education courses;

- reduced-rate tuition for academic courses;

- bookstore gift certificates;

- adjunct or affiliate faculty appointment;

- differential pay or adjustment of work schedule (e.g., exemption from weekend shifts) for preceptors who work with new staff members;

- a gift such as a fruit basket or plant (Bain, 1996; Jackson, 2001; LeGris & Côte, 1997).

SUMMARY

The use of preceptors is an alternative to the traditional clinical teaching model based on the assumption that a consistent relationship between an experienced nurse and a nursing student or novice staff nurse is an effective method of providing individualized guidance in clinical learning and professional socialization. Preceptorships have been used extensively with senior nursing students, graduate students preparing for advanced practice roles, and new staff nurse orientees.

A preceptorship is a time-limited, one-to-one relationship between a learner and an experienced nurse. The teacher is not physically present during the clinical learning activities; the preceptor provides intensive, individualized learning opportunities that improve the learner's clinical competence and confidence. The teacher has overall responsibility for the quality of the clinical teaching and learning and provides the link between the educational program and the practice setting. The preceptor functions as a role model and provides individualized clinical instruction, support, and socialization for the learner.

Preceptorships are frequently used for students in their last semester of academic preparation for entry into practice, and for graduate students preparing for advanced clinical practice, administration, and education roles. In many health care organizations, preceptors participate in the orientation of newly hired staff nurses by acting as role models and supporting new staff members' professional socialization.

The use of preceptors in clinical teaching has both advantages and disadvantages for the preceptors, clinical agencies, students, and educational program. Benefits for preceptors and their employers include the stimulation of working with learners who raise questions about clinical practice, assistance from students with research or teaching projects, rewards through a clinical ladder system for participation as a preceptor, and opportunities to recruit potential staff members for the agency from among students who work with preceptors. The greatest drawback of preceptorships to agencies and preceptors usually is the expected time commitment.

Students experience the benefits of working one-on-one with clinical experts who can coach them to improved performance as well as opportunities to experience the realities of clinical practice. However, following their preceptors' schedules often creates conflicts with students' academic, work, and family commitments.

Preceptorships offer many advantages to teachers and educational programs. The use of preceptors provides more clinical teachers for students and thus more intensive guidance of students' learning activities. Working collaboratively with preceptors also helps faculty members to stay informed about the current realities of practice. Disadvantages include the amount of indirect teaching time required to select, prepare, and communicate with preceptors and students.

Selection of appropriate preceptors is important to the success of preceptorships. Most academic programs require the preceptor to have at least the degree for which the student is preparing. Desire to teach and willingness to serve as a preceptor are very important qualities of potential preceptors. Additional attributes of effective preceptors include clinical expertise or proficiency, leadership abilities, teaching skill, and professional role behaviors and attitudes.

Teachers are responsible for initial orientation and continuing support of all participants; preparation can be formal or informal. A general orientation for potential preceptors may include information about benefits and challenges of precepting, characteristics of a good preceptor, principles of adult learning, clinical teaching and evaluation methods, and the structure and goals of the nursing education program. After preceptors have been selected, they need a specific orientation to their responsibilities, including information about the educational level and previous experience of the student, choosing specific learning activities based on learning objectives, and scheduling of clinical learning activities. Learners also need an orientation that includes the purposes of the preceptorship, the process of planning individual learning activities, and an explanation of teacher and preceptor roles.

Successful implementation of preceptorships depends on mutual understanding of the roles and responsibilities of the participants. The preceptor is expected to be a positive role model and a resource person for the student. The responsibilities of the preceptor include creating a positive learning climate, including the student in activities that relate to learning goals, and providing feedback to the student and teacher. The student usually arranges the schedule of clinical learning activities to coincide with the preceptor's work schedule and is expected to participate actively in planning learning activities. Because the teacher is not always present during learning activities, the student must keep the teacher informed about progress through frequent communication. In addition to making preceptor selections and orienting preceptors and students, the teacher is an important resource to preceptors and students to assist in problem solving. Teachers must make adequate arrangements for communication with other participants.

A common strategy for planning and implementing students' learning activities is the use of an individualized learning contract, an explicit agreement among teacher, student, and preceptor that specifies the learning goals, learning activities selected to meet the objectives, and the expected outcomes and criteria by which they will be evaluated. The learning contract serves as a guide for planning and implementing the student's learning activities.

Students, teachers, and preceptors share responsibility for monitoring the progress of learning and for evaluating outcomes of the preceptorship. Student performance is assessed according to the terms specified in the learning contract or through the clinical evaluation methods used by the educational program, through self-evaluation, and through feedback from preceptors. The teacher is responsible for the summative evaluation of learner performance. Students are an important source of information about their preceptors' clinical teaching effectiveness, but the teacher should also assess the degree to which preceptors were able to effectively guide students' learning.

Preceptors should receive appropriate rewards and incentives for the contributions they make to the educational program. At minimum, every preceptor should receive an individualized thank-you letter, specifying some of the benefits that the student received from the preceptorship. Other formal and informal ways of acknowledging the contributions of preceptors were discussed.

REFERENCES

Bain, L. (1996). Preceptorship: A review of the literature. *Journal of Advanced Nursing, 24,* 104–107.

Case, B., & Oermann, M. H. (2004). Teaching in a clinical setting. In L. Caputi & L. Engelmann (Eds.), *Teaching nursing: The art and science* (pp. 126–177). Glen Ellyn, IL: College of DuPage Press.

Hardy, R., & Smith, R. (2001). Enhancing staff development with a structured preceptor program. *Journal of Nursing Care Quality, 15,* 9–17.

Jackson, M. (2001). A preceptor incentive program. *American Journal of Nursing, 101,* 24A–24E.

Kersbergen, A. L., & Hrobsky, P. E. (1996). Use of clinical map guides in precepted clinical experiences. *Nurse Educator, 21,* 19–22.

LeGris, J., & Côte, F. H. (1997). Collaborative partners in nursing education: A preceptorship model for BscN students. *Nursing Connections, 10,* 55–70.

Mamchur, C., & Myrick, F. (2003) Preceptorship and interpersonal conflict: A multidisciplinary study. *Journal of Advanced Nursing, 43,* 188–196.

Myrick, F., & Yonge, O. (2002). Preceptor behaviors integral to the promotion of critical thinking ability of baccalaureate students in the practice setting. *Journal for Nurses in Staff Development, 18,* 127–133.

Myrick, F., & Yonge, O. (2003). Preceptorship: A quintessential component of nursing education. In M. H. Oermann & K. T. Heinrich (Eds.), *Annual review of nursing education* (Vol. 1, pp. 91–107). New York: Springer Publishing.

Nordgren, J., Richardson, S. J., & Laurella, V. B. (1998). A collaborative preceptor model for clinical teaching of beginning nursing students. *Nurse Educator, 23,* 27–32.

Stokes, L., & Kost, G. (2005). Teaching in the clinical setting. In D. M. Billings & J. A. Halstead (Eds.), *Teaching in nursing: A guide for faculty* (2nd ed., pp. 325–348). St. Louis: Elsevier Saunders.

Yonge, O., Myrick, F., & Haase, M. (2002). Student nurse stress in the preceptorship experience. *Nurse Educator, 27,* 84–88.

Chapter 15

Clinical Teaching in Diverse Settings

Diane M. Wink

Nursing care occurs in diverse settings—multiple types of health care and non–health care locations where there are clients (individuals, families, communities) who can benefit from the services of a professional nurse. Professional nurses take on multiple roles as they work with clients of all ages, races, ethnic groups, and cultures. These clients have the full scope of health promotion, health maintenance, and acute, chronic, and rehabilitation care needs.

In an ideal world, all nursing students would have clinical learning activities in all settings, with all client groups, and in all professional nursing roles. In addition to preparation for the challenges of nursing practice today, students would be prepared to adapt to the change as clients, health issues, care locations, and approaches to care evolve. Students would have opportunities to work with clients from cultures other than their own and implement care that recognizes the global influences on both health and illness.

Nurse educators and their students do not live in an ideal world. All students cannot participate in all of these learning activities during their nursing education. Choices must be made with the hope that the breadth and depth of students' clinical learning activities result in the development of the core competencies and skills needed for safe and effective nursing practice. For students who are already nurses, their clinical experiences must help them grow as professionals as they move to more advanced levels of practice.

Traditionally, much of clinical nursing education takes place in acute care settings because of long-held assumptions about how nurses must be prepared to practice. These assumptions include the beliefs that traditional inpatient settings are the best sites for learning essential clinical knowledge; acute-care skills are the most important skills to learn; a prescribed sequence of specialty clinical rotations is required; and faculty members must directly oversee student activities to ensure student learning and evaluate skills (Ryan, D'Aoust, Groth, McGee, & Small, 1997). Traditional settings for the clinical education of nursing students include primarily hospital units that provide care to adults in addition to selected community-based health care agencies such as home care and public health agencies. Because of decreasing length of inpatient stays and economic pressures to provide care in outpatient and community settings, limited (and in some cases decreased) numbers of clinical learning activities take place on units that provide care for children, individuals with psychiatric illnesses, and women and families during pregnancy and childbirth.

The realities in traditional acute-care settings make many clinical learning opportunities located there suboptimal. Clients have increasingly complex illnesses and receive high-technology interventions in an attempt to repair, cure, or ameliorate illness and injury. Because of this high patient acuity and complexity, many sites do not allow for achievement of the full scope of clinical learning objectives. Collaboration with other disciplines, acting as a change agent, being a patient advocate, and even development of many key assessment and psychomotor skills can be difficult in a setting where all clients are critically ill. And, because of the increasingly specialized nature of many acute care units (e.g., cardiovascular, orthopedic, endocrine) it is hard for students to see a broad scope of client problems when they have a finite number of clinical hours and a predetermined schedule. The use of diverse care sites is essential if students are to achieve all course and program objectives (Tanner, 2006).

Even when traditional acute-care placements are appropriate, implementing clinical learning activities in such settings can be challenging. High demand for placements from nursing education programs (often with rapidly increasing enrollments) and other health professional programs has overwhelmed many acute-care agencies. Both staff members and patients can be asked to interact with students 24 hours a day, 7 days a week. As a result, acute-care agencies often place limitations on the numbers of students per unit or the days and times that students can be present. In some cases, the mandated clinical group size is so limited that some students in a clinical group must be scheduled for observation activities elsewhere so that fewer students are on the unit, or the group size has to be kept very small, a remedy that usually is not economically feasible for the nursing education program.

However, the presence of nurses and the need for nursing care in locations other than acute care is well known. Today, patients outside of acute-care institutions are sicker and have increased needs for nursing care. As the patients and nurses have moved out of acute-care settings, so have the clinical learning opportunities. Thus while surgery once was performed almost exclusively in hospitals, many clients now have procedures in freestanding surgical centers. Patients once spent weeks recovering in hospitals after surgery or while recovering from trauma; they now recover at rehabilitation facilities or at home. No longer are patients who need long-term parenteral therapy or antibiotics kept in an inpatient facility. Full management of their care is carried out by nurses working in rehabilitation, long-term care, and home health settings.

Community-based nursing occurs wherever and whenever nurses work in collaboration with the client and community as part of interdisciplinary and intra-disciplinary teams to provide care across the continuum (Matteson, 2000). How-ever, community-health nursing (CHN), or public health nursing, is a process of delivering nursing care to improve the health of a community. Individuals may be recipients of care, but the focus is on the total community, especially high-risk ag-gregates (Zotti, Brown, & Stotts, 1996).

CLINICAL LEARNING ACTIVITIES IN DIVERSE SETTINGS

Nursing care can be learned wherever students have contact with clients. Learn-ing objectives do not prescribe a specific setting where the learning activities must take place. The core components of a clinical learning activity—including client contact; opportunities for students to have an active role in client assessment, goal setting, and then planning, implementing, and evaluating care; critical-thinking and problem-solving opportunities; competent guidance (from the teacher or some-one designated to take on the teaching role in that site); and skill development (in-tellectual as well as psychomotor)—can be present even in settings other than acute-care hospital units.

Placement of nursing students in diverse clinical settings has multiple bene-fits. These include preparing the student to be a part of the health care system in which the acute-care hospital is but one part. Not only will students learn about these sites, they will develop the skills that these settings are best able to provide. For example, development of a psychomotor skill such as initiation of intravenous therapy and the many clinical assessment and decision-making skills that go with this routine procedure may best take place in a perioperative setting. Development of therapeutic communication competencies may be best achieved in rehabilita-tion settings where it is possible to have client contact over time. Care planning, evaluation, and revision may be best developed in a home health setting where care planning is fully integrated into client services. The home health setting also lends itself to development of collaboration skills as well as real-world knowledge about the impact of payer status and insurance reimbursement on the ability of the client to pay for (and in many cases receive) needed care.

Clinical learning activities in community-based settings allow nursing students to work with clients where the clients live and work. Students see the challenges that clients face as they implement self-care for health promotion and maintenance as well as care for their own and family members' acute and chronic illnesses. Collaboration with other members of the health care team is a natural, necessary, and active part of care delivery in community-based settings.

Nursing students can participate in creatively designed, rigorous high-quality clinical leaning activities almost any place. This chapter gives examples of diverse clinical learning activities, reviews some of the practical aspects of implementing clinical learning activities in diverse settings, addresses problems commonly faced in these placements, and suggests solutions for such problems.

EXAMPLES OF DIVERSE SETTINGS FOR CLINICAL LEARNING ACTIVITIES

Clinical learning activities in diverse settings include opportunities for students to meet specific learning objectives while caring for clients. Three categories are used as examples of such activities. The first consists of patient care areas that are not regularly used as clinical learning sites. Some of these (e.g., the operating room) have been virtually eliminated as clinical learning sites in most nursing programs, while others (e.g., outpatient clinics, nursing homes) are underused, despite the rich learning opportunities provided for students in these settings. The second category includes sites where provision of health care is not the prime focus of the site or agency. Examples are schools, camps, congregate meal sites, senior citizen programs, and apartment complexes. These sites may be extensively used in community-based nursing education curricula but can provide excellent clinical learning opportunities in all programs. Some of these activities may be service-learning experiences if they reflect key components of service-learning. See Chapter 7 for information on planning high-quality service-learning activities. The third category is the growing use of international clinical learning opportunities. These can be brief (often 1 week) placements in which students are part of a team providing a continuum of health services, or extended placements in which the student lives for weeks to months in the country in which the clinical activities are based.

There are other clinical learning activities not included in this discussion. One is an observation, in which students' objectives are best achieved while they maintain a nonparticipant role in the clinical setting. Another is a special event held as part of a clinical rotation, such as a trip to an art gallery or to attend a play, designed to help students increase a specific skill, competency, or self-awareness. Clinical observations and interactions that are part of a didactic course also are not included. While potentially valuable as learning activities, riding in an ambulance with emergency medical service providers or visiting a hospital, clinic, or client group as part of a course (whether at home or in another country) is a not a clinical learning activity if there is no client care in which the student participates.

Clinical Learning in Underused Patient Care Sites

With the diversity of clinical practice sites, there are many examples of clinical learning activities. Several are used here to illustrate how such sites can be optimized.

Outpatient Clinics.   Outpatient settings such as primary care practices, specialty clinics, and rehabilitation programs often are difficult to use effectively as clinical learning sites because of the lack of RN role models and the difficulty of placing large numbers of students at one site, making clinical teaching by the faculty difficult. These problems can be addressed through placement of students in a single large clinical facility.

For example, in a community-based course that focused on development of assessment, client problem identification, and family-centered care, a nursing student group was placed at a Veterans Administration clinic. The site had multiple specialty and internal medicine clinics each with a team of professionals who worked collaboratively with the other specialty teams. RNs in this clinic were responsible for basic client assessment as well as education and follow-up after provider visits. The RNs interacted with a wide range of providers such as nurse practitioners, physician's assistants, and family practice and specialty physicians, as well as the clients and their families.

After orientation to the site, students rotated among the specialty clinics. The instructor was able to be on-site throughout the clinical learning activity because the size of the clinic accommodated the entire student group. Students changed specialty clinics each week but the common staff and assessment tools, the fact that the providers (NPs, physicians, nurses, social workers) all worked in the same system, and the common client population made the transition smooth.

Regular student–faculty conferences allowed review of the challenges faced by clients and families that the students identified. Students also discussed patterns in assessment findings and interventions to address their ongoing health promotion and maintenance needs of the clients. Because of the wide range of health problems among the clients, content from the accompanying didactic courses was constantly reinforced. The students developed a rich array of skills including completing health histories, focused physical assessments, administration of medications, and collaboration with families and other members of the health care team. They also gained an in-depth knowledge of a major subset of our health care system (B. Gross, personal communication, November, 2005).

Operating Room.   Most nursing education programs eliminated an operating room (OR) clinical rotation from their curricula many years ago, but in doing so, nursing faculties have overlooked many rich clinical learning opportunities. Many of the hospitalized clients for whom acute-care nurses provide care pass through the OR at some time in their hospitalization. Knowledge about patients' surgical experiences can greatly enhance the knowledge and skill of the nurse caring for the patients both before and after surgery.

AORN, the Association of periOperative Registered Nurses, has issued a position statement encouraging nursing education programs to increase use of perioperative settings as clinical learning sites. AORN proposed that the perioperative environment is an ideal setting for teaching application of the nursing process and that perioperative clinical learning activities can contribute to the achievement of a wide variety of program outcomes. Because of the current emphasis on patient safety, perioperative settings offer opportunities to study human factors and communication theories. Perioperative clinical learning activities can be integrated into any nursing curriculum (AORN, 2006).

Nursing students can develop a wide array of psychomotor skills in perioperative settings, such as catheter care, insertion and maintenance of intravenous lines, pain management, skin and wound care, and care of unconscious patients. A series of perioperative learning activities across the curriculum can help nursing education programs produce learning outcomes required to achieve and maintain accreditation (Sigsby, 2004). In addition, inclusion of perioperative learning activities in undergraduate nursing curricula will increase nurses' knowledge of clients' surgical experiences, regardless of setting in which the nurses work, and may increase the number of nursing students who choose the perioperative specialty after graduation (Mitchell, Stevens, Goodman, & Brown, 2002; Sigsby & Yarandi, 2004).

In one study, knowledge of topics related to the nursing care of surgical patients (e.g., aseptic technique, safety, infection control, medication administration, and legal and ethical aspects of informed consent) was compared among students in a medical-surgical clinical course with and without a perioperative rotation. This knowledge was found to be equivalent or greater among students who had the perioperative rotation (Sigsby & Yarandi, 2004).

Another way to include more perioperative clinical learning activities is with an elective course in perioperative nursing, such as the one created by the partnership of St. Luke's Hospital and Prairie View University. Students had concentrated didactic content followed by clinical learning activities and a lecture each week. Students performed the scrub role with staff members and had specific objectives for each week that reflected their knowledge and skill development. Conference time was a part of the learning activities as well as formal patient care planning (Mitchell, et al., 2002).

Faculty members at Clayton College and State University worked with the local AORN chapter and the staff and administration at a local OR to develop an elective course in perioperative nursing. The course was offered in the summer term between the junior and senior year. In addition to completing didactic coursework on topics such as patient safety, collaboration, anesthesia, prevention of complications, and legal aspects of perioperative nursing, students were placed with staff preceptors in the clinical component of the program. Several students were able to have additional perioperative nursing experiences in subsequent rotations and several expressed interest in working in a perioperative setting after graduation (Kurtz & Eichelberger, 1999).

Nursing Home.   Competency in the care of older adults, including frail elders, is a desired outcome of all nursing curricula. Almost all graduates will be caring for elderly clients regardless of work setting.

An underused clinical learning setting for gaining these competencies is the nursing home. Nursing homes provide an opportunity for students to practice multiple psychomotor skills and learn to provide long-term care to a single client. In this setting, observation of changes over time is possible while caring for clients with complex needs. But due to the stable nature of nursing home clients' health problems, nursing students are not likely to be overwhelmed by the complexity of the care. With a rich variety of clients, learning needs can be matched with clinical learning assignments as students provide holistic care over a full range of physical, psychological, spiritual, environmental, and financial areas (Chen, Melcher, Witucki, & McKibben, 2002). Nursing homes provide many opportunities for students to practice implementing care that has a long-term impact. Bowel and urinary continence programs, programs to improve nutrition, and interventions to increase social interaction are a few examples of such activities.

Another benefit of student clinical learning activities in nursing homes is their role in improvement of care for the residents of the facility. Faculty members can serve as clinical experts and role models, and students have the time needed to implement and support programs that help clients achieve objectives hard to reach in today's health care environment. The Texas Tech University Health Sciences Center faculty revised its curriculum to better integrate content on the care of older adults based on the work of the Hartford Foundation for Geriatric Nursing. A 30-hour practicum in long-term care was made part of a larger 3-credit hour clinical course taken in the senior year. Faculty members collaborate with a long-term care facility to create a "Teaching Nursing Home" experience. Students collaborate with a clinical preceptor to complete a variety of activities at the nursing home. These include targeted psychological and physiological assessments of residents and the use of the Minimum Data Set for Long-term Care as well as review and assessment of client data in individual records. Analysis of the data and comparison of student assessments to data in the client records is another learning activity. The students also take an active role in the case management of selected clients.

There are some barriers to high-quality clinical learning experiences in nursing homes. One is the lack of nursing role models. Faculty members can overcome this deficiency by being role models themselves. In addition, students can use this opportunity to improve collaboration skills as they work with the wide variety of supportive staff from nursing assistants, LPNs, RNs, physical therapists and occupational therapists, nutrition staff, and administrators. Negative attitudes of students toward elderly clients, either preexisting or as a result of the nursing home experience, are another concern. Again, the attitudes and approach of the faculty member can help prevent or address this issue (Chen et al., 2002).

Hospice.   Competency in delivering end-of-life care is another of the expected student outcomes of nursing education. This competency can be difficult to achieve in classic clinical settings where students have limited exposure and opportunity to interact with dying clients and their families. A clinical learning activity in a hospice is an excellent way both to expose students to the issues related to end-of-life care as well as to develop many skills needed in all nursing roles and settings. For example, faculty members at one college developed a program in which students were teamed with a hospice worker to follow families receiving hospice services during an 8-week mental health course. Faculty members identified multiple course goals as well as American Association of Colleges of Nursing (AACN) and End-of-Life Nursing Education Consortium (ELNEC) competencies that would be met through this activity. These included development of effective and compassionate communication skills with the client, family, and team members; recognition of students' own attitudes and feelings about death; and demonstration of respect for the family while assisting them through end-of-life care.

Students met weekly with their assigned family with the support of both the course faculty and a hospice team member. Students were instructed to tell the families the length of time they would be working with them and that the students were there to talk about anything the clients or families wanted to speak about. Weekly support groups with faculty members and peers offered additional assistance to students as they addressed issues and emotions of clients, families, and students that arose during this clinical learning activity. Evaluation of the learning activity was overwhelmingly positive and achievement of AACN competencies was clear (Hayes, 2005).

Crisis Center.   Agencies that care for psychiatric clients outside of acute-care institutions now are the backbone of psychiatric care. They also offer rich clinical learning opportunities. DeLashmutt and Rankin (2005) described use of a crisis center during a psychiatric mental health clinical course developed to increase students' knowledge and understanding of poverty. Students spent 4 days of a semester-long psychiatric-mental health clinical course at a crisis-focused day shelter and multi-resource advocacy center for poor and homeless individuals and families. Students completed specific reading and audiovisual assignments to support the clinical learning activity. There also were four focused postclinical conference discussions on the lived experience of mental illness, homelessness, feminization of poverty, and integration of concepts related to the clinical learning activity. In two of the conferences, guests such as a homeless individual or a formerly homeless mentally ill mother joined the students. Outcomes of the experience were examined using a pre- and postexperience questionnaire. Responses demonstrated that the students had experienced both personal and professional growth. The structured postclinical conferences contributed to this growth.

Community-Based Clinical Learning Activities

Almost all clients cared for by nurses in the acute care setting come from and return to the community. In addition, there are many issues, particularly related to health promotion and maintenance and care of chronic disease, which are best addressed in community settings. Community settings also offer many learning opportunities for development of key skills and competencies that are hard to meet in the very intense acute-care environment. For these reasons, inclusion of community-based clinical learning activities in the nursing curriculum is important.

Community-based experiences are often implemented under the umbrella of service-learning. In service-learning, students work collaboratively with community partners to meet both course and community objectives. Reflection on the experience and development of a sense of civic engagement are essential components. (See Chapter 7 for a more in-depth discussion of service-learning.)

In many nursing education programs, often those with community-based curricula, students have clinical learning activities in a wide variety of agencies in a single community or geographic area. Students in community-based programs return to the community repeatedly during their nursing education and often have a final culminating project designed to address a specific health care need of the community (Kiehl & Wink, 2000; Matteson, 1995, 2000; Wink, 2003).

In a study of associate degree and baccalaureate nursing programs with community-based experiences, programs reported student clinical placements in a wide variety of settings. These included health departments, schools, home health agencies, and prisons. Students completed a wide variety of nursing interventions including administration of immunizations and disease surveillance. It was not uncommon for students to work independently (with a faculty member making site visits) or under the supervision of preceptors part of the time (Frank, Adams, Edelstein, Speakman, & Shelton, 2005).

Two projects exemplifying how such activities can achieve both course and curricular objectives were implemented by students at the University of Central Florida. A homeless shelter was the clinical learning site for a small group of students who provided basic health screenings, referrals, and education in a clinical rotation in their junior year. In addition to learning about issues of homelessness, the students developed relationships with the residents and staff, honed their health history and physical assessment skills, and increased their knowledge of the chronic and acute physical and mental health problems of shelter residents. As a result, students identified a need for a program for the children in the shelter, focusing on grief and loss. The students developed a program for the children that interpreted these concepts broadly to include loss of home, friends, and family as well as loss from death. In addition, during the presentation of the grief program, multiple episodes of pets dying or running away surfaced as a form of loss.

An elementary school was the clinical learning site for a group of students who helped complete the yearly state-mandated assessments, again as part of a clinical rotation in their junior year. Assessments included blood pressure (BP), height, weight, body mass index (BMI) (interpreted based on the child's age), and vision, hearing, and scoliosis screening. Using course objectives and principles of primary, secondary, and tertiary prevention as guides, the students learned how to complete the assessments correctly, work with children of varied ages, analyze their findings, and identify problems that they as students could help the school's staff address over the next year.

In their final semester, these students implemented a case management project in which children identified as overweight were further assessed. The students developed tools needed to track the children and communicate with the parents and (with permission) the child's health care providers. Educational and support programs were offered to both the children and parents. Primary prevention was implemented through an educational project on fitness and nutrition, secondary prevention included the screening of all the children, and the tertiary prevention focus was the BP project. Nursing students measured the BP of any child with a BMI at or above the 85th percentile. The students used a case management approach, wrote a referral letter to the parents, and reported outcomes to the health department from which they had secured permission to do the BP project (I. Sheplan, personal communication, February 3, 2006).

Community-based learning activities are not limited to baccalaureate programs; they can occur in associate degree programs also (Tagliareni & Speakman, 2003). Ligeikis-Clayton and Denman (2005) described a multisemester program in a community college in which students were placed with one of 15 agencies with four to six students per site. A service-learning coordinator visited the sites, developed contracts, and managed the program. Nursing faculty members served as liaison for one or two agencies each, with contact at least once a semester. The clinical hours for the project were hours previously used for observational community activities. Agency preceptors helped the students learn about the agency and its purpose and challenges and worked with the students to identify projects and then carry them out. The service-learning projects were discussed in postclinical conferences throughout the four semesters of the program.

Camps.   Another community-based site that can meet many clinical learning objectives, particularly those related to the care of children with acute and chronic illnesses, is a camp. Use of summer camps for children for the clinical component of a community health course was described by Toften and Fonnesbeck (2002). The clinical learning activity took place in a camp of the student's choice: traditional, special needs, or underprivileged youths.

In addition to the camp activities themselves, students had opportunities to assess and treat children with hydration, sleep, nutrition, and communicable disease issues. They also learned about and then used the public health resources and local community agencies that helped them address the public health, environmental, and psychomotor needs of the children. To meet the community health objectives of the clinical learning activity, students completed a community assessment of the camp, its clients, and the surrounding community. Students worked with the camp staff to identify a needed project that could be the focus of student work at the camps. Because this was an ongoing program, projects were often the result of assessments initiated the year before (Toften & Fonnesbeck, 2002).

Child Care Centers.   Child care centers offer many opportunities for students to develop observation, developmental assessment, physical assessment, and teaching skills. Goetz and Nissen (2005) reported on use of a day care center as one of many sites during the clinical component of an introductory associate degree nursing program course focused on assessment of different age groups. The students were placed at the center for 2 days to meet specific objectives related to communication with children, assessment, and analysis of the child's physical and developmental status. Each student focused on one child per day and completed a well-child assessment under the direct observation of the instructor. All students also did teaching projects as small groups and participated in conferences in which they analyzed their observations and discussed how they had to modify approaches based on the unique characteristics of each child.

Use of a variety of community locations for a single clinical course in pediatric nursing practice was described by Hitt and Overbay (1997). A combination of sites was used to provide pediatric clinical learning activities based on a model of primary, secondary, and tertiary health promotion. Required activities related to all three levels of health promotion; enrichment activities provided in-depth opportunities to meet individual learning needs and interests. Required primary health promotion activities took place in day care centers and preschools; enrichment activities were offered in a high school and at a health screening for home-schooled children. Required secondary health promotion activities in the community hospital pediatric unit allowed students to focus on care of the child with health deviations and the effect of the illness on the child and family; enrichment activities were offered at a burn unit, a pediatric intensive care unit, and an ambulatory surgery unit. The focus of tertiary health promotion activities was on the child with a chronic or terminal illness. Required learning activities were located in a pediatric rehabilitation hospital and a pediatric long-term care facility; enrichment activities included extended opportunities in either of these facilities or making home visits to pediatric patients with a home health care nurse.

Senior Housing.   Arrington (1997) suggested that nursing education programs located in areas with large retirement communities have a rich source of potential clinical sites. A retirement community includes residents with a variety of lifestyles, physical abilities, and interests, and therefore provides opportunities for nursing students to assess the comorbidities and differences among individuals in an aging population. In this account of the use of a retirement community as a clinical site, nursing students participated in clinical learning activities under the guidance of a certified gerontological nurse in the position of health consultant who provided health promotion and health maintenance services. Learning objectives focused on developing communication and basic psychomotor skills; assessing mobility, safety concerns, vision and hearing deficits, and mental status; health education; and developing positive attitudes about the aging process.

Graduate-Level Community-Based Clinical Activities.   At the graduate level, the focus of clinical placements is often on the specific clinical specialization for which the student is being prepared. However, students also must learn how to collect and use community- and practice-based data that identify needed changes in practice structure and function to better care for the communities, families, and individuals served by their practice. The ability to plan, implement, and evaluate outcomes of changes is also essential.

Programs and facilities for homeless individuals and families provided clinical learning sites for graduate nursing students in an entry-level master's program described by Wolf, Goldfader, and Lehan (1997). Objectives included learning population-focused health promotion and communicating with people for whom trust and acceptance were challenging. Learning activities included performing a community assessment of an urban homeless community; assessing and providing care to homeless people in drop-in and day care programs, individual and family shelters, and a foot clinic for substance-abusing homeless men and women; and providing homeless women with opportunities for self-expression through a writing project. Students learned a broad definition of primary care and creative approaches to person-centered care.

An effective option for achieving desired learning outcomes is to incorporate practice at diverse sites (often sites where it is difficult or inappropriate for the students to do a formal or full clinical rotation) through service-learning activities. Graduate students can collaborate with community partners during which students meet course objectives while helping the community partner (e.g., a practice site) meet mutually agreed on objectives. As a part of the process, students have an opportunity to reflect on their experiences and the relationship between the community and their learning.

At the University of Central Florida, Master of Science in Nursing students in the nurse practitioner (NP) tracks work in small groups to complete a two-semester service-learning project to address problems and issues identified by community partners. In one project, the NP students worked with a multisite clinic for uninsured, low-income individuals to assess the effectiveness of its procedures for communicating lab and diagnostic test results to patients. Their findings led to a revision in the clinic's procedures and tools that addressed unique situations at its different sites.

Another graduate student group worked with a local hospital and community providers across the area on strategies to improve follow-up care of patients recovering from a stroke. The students developed tools to improve communication about needed care and implemented several educational programs for both providers and patients. Despite the formal end of the project, two of the students continued to disseminate the tools in the community. One set up a poststroke follow-up program in the primary care where he was later employed.

A third group worked with a federally qualified health clinic to audit charts of clients being treated for hypertension to determine how well providers met standards of care. Several deficiencies were identified and addressed via staff education and changes in procedure. In all these cases, the community partner gained much needed expertise in the development or evaluation of programs essential to their mission and the students had an opportunity to see the health care system from the inside, particularly trying to meet the needs of the uninsured and underinsured.

In another example, advanced practice nurse faculty members used two nurse-managed wellness centers as clinical learning sites (Resick, Taylor, Carroll, D'Antonio, & de Chesnay, 1997; Taylor, Resick, D'Antonio, & Carroll, 1997). Nurse-managed wellness clinics established in two urban elderly high-rise apartment buildings provided opportunities for faculty practice as well as clinical learning sites for undergraduate and graduate students in nursing, pharmacy, and

occupational therapy. Learning activities varied according to the student's educational level and discipline, and included health assessment, environmental assessment, health education, monitoring of chronic health problems, and support
for self-care. These activities enabled students to meet learning objectives related
to a wellness and health promotion model of care for elderly persons; promoting
health, functioning, and quality of life for older adults; and developing positive attitudes toward elderly individuals. Graduate students preparing for roles as advanced practice nurses also benefited from the role modeling of the wellness center
nurse managers.

International Sites

Clinical placements in international sites can be rich opportunities that expand
students' comfort and competence in care of diverse clients beyond that which
can be gained in course work focusing on such content. Learning activities that
take place within the students' own culture and familiar surroundings do not always help students meet goals relating to becoming culturally sensitive because
the clients' worldviews do not predominate (Kavanagh, 1998). Clinical learning
sites in international health settings can help students develop cultural sensitivity and competence as well as a global view of nursing and health care (Oneha,
Magnussen, & Feletti, 1998). Nursing students whose clinical activities take place
within other cultures, in both developed and developing countries, are challenged
intellectually and emotionally, and must learn to manage culture shock (Kavanagh,
1998).

Caffrey, Neander, Markle, and Stewart (2005) compared 32 undergraduate
nursing students using the Caffrey Cultural Competence in Healthcare Scale. All
students had classes that integrated cultural content. A small subset of the group
(7 students) also had a 5-week immersion experience working in a nursing role in
Guatemala. Student self-perceived knowledge and comfort with skills showed little
change among those who had only the didactic content. However, the students
who had the immersion experience had very large increases in all areas. While the
authors acknowledged the impact of self-selection to participate in the immersion
experience on the results, they also found no differences in scores of the two groups
on pretesting. Differences did not appear until after the clinical work in the international setting was completed (Caffrey et al., 2005).

A long-term view of the impact of an international clinical placement was
provided by Duffy, Farmer, Ravert, and Huittinen (2005). They surveyed students
2 years after an international placement. The former participants in international
placements reported a continued positive impact on their professional and personal lives as well as increased cultural sensitivity. The specific nature of the

international experience was found to make a difference in the nature of student response. Students reported concerns common to all clinical learning activities (e.g., fear of error and the unknown; not being familiar with the patient, patient problems, the agency, and agency policies). However, the students also showed a progression in their knowledge and understanding of the other country and health care system as they moved from what the investigators called a "micro to a macro" view. The students began to see the bigger picture and how both nursing care and the health care system functioned.

There is some evidence that student growth is greater after experiences in developing countries as compared to those in developed countries, although there is overall growth regardless of the nature of the placement (Thompson, Boore, & Deeny, 2000). In an extensive review of the literature on international placements, Button, Green, Tengnah, Johansson, and Baker (2005) found four benefits: learning cultural differences, comparing health care systems, comparing nursing practice, and personal development.

Regardless of the site or nature of the experience, the inherent limitations of student learning activities in other cultures must be considered. Even after a long-term experience in another country, can a person actually become "culturally competent?" Can someone actually understand the complexities of another culture? Is not a true understanding of a culture an evolving process that takes place over many years and extensive experience (Crigger & Holcomb, in press)?

Students must also be helped to comprehend how even the most generous care can result in harm to those they are working with. Inappropriate use of antibiotics and provision of care and interventions that cannot be sustained after the team departs are not appropriate, however well-meaning (Crigger & Holcomb, in press). When working in developing countries and any setting without a strong formal health care system, the World Health Organization (2002) principles of rational prescribing must be considered:

> Patients receive medications appropriate to their clinical needs, in doses that meet their own individual requirements for an adequate period of time, and at the lowest cost to them and their community.

Preparation for clinical learning activities in other countries is essential, including student understanding of the environment and health care system in which they will be placed. Students need to be prepared for the fact that nursing practice as well as the settings for that care will be different. An understanding of the overall culture, communication patterns, values of the community and country in which they will be placed, and knowledge of the health care system of that country and community is also essential. Even with extensive preparation, and whether the student goes to a developed or developing country, support from peers and faculty and an opportunity to debrief are needed (Button et al., 2005; Grant & McKenna, 2003).

Many practical aspects of learning activities at international sites also must be addressed. The source institution for the nursing education program may have an international placement office that can assist with arrangements. Completion of necessary paperwork for that office staff is essential. Such paperwork usually includes a waiver of responsibility of the source educational institution and a separate application for the international activity. Students also must be informed of costs, which usually include tuition for the course, transportation, housing and food costs at the site, and cost of day-to-day expenses, including local travel. Additional insurance for emergency health care and travel back home may be needed. Depending on the host country and type of site, verification of licensure of graduate nursing students and accompanying faculty members and protocols to cover any nursing care to be delivered by them may be needed.

Students will need passports with an expiration date well beyond the end of the planned learning activity. Additional immunizations are often required. Most immunization series must be started well in advance of the planned trip. Some trips, particularly those in developing countries, rural areas, or locations at higher altitudes than students' country of origin, may require physical conditioning as well.

Practical aspects of life at the distant site must also be addressed. These include appropriate clothing for clinical activities. What does a nurse or volunteer health care provider wear in the host country? What equipment will the student need to provide? For mission trips in which the group will not be placed at a permanent health care site, are there materials that the students are expected to help gather or transport? Preparation for the day-to-day living conditions, including food and water safety, is essential. Housing should also be considered. Will the students be housed in a hotel, home, dormitory, or tent? Is there a choice? Education related to personal safety including both health and environmental risks is essential.

Emergency planning is also essential. This planning includes what to do if a student becomes separated from the group as well as a frank discussion of what students and faculty members should do if there should be a natural disaster or act of war or terrorism. Where should they go? When? Whom should they contact and how can that contact be completed?

Many international placements are a part of an ongoing partnership. For example, two university schools of nursing have reported relationships with schools in Nicaragua (Riner & Becklenberg, 2001; Ross, 1998).

Collaboration between these U.S. universities and their Nicaraguan counterparts produced outcomes such as student and faculty exchange activities focused on community and acute health care, and development of an elective course for the U.S. nursing students. International clinical learning activities enabled U.S.

nursing students to meet objectives of providing holistic care to culturally diverse populations.

PRACTICAL ASPECTS OF CLINICAL PLACEMENTS IN DIVERSE SITES

When looking at practical aspects of clinical placements in diverse sites, there are two major areas of concern. The first includes the regulatory and accreditation requirements for clinical learning activities; the second is preparation of the agency, faculty, and students.

Regulatory and Accreditation Requirements

All clinical learning activities must meet requirements of state law and regulations (often set by the board of nursing) as well as the policies and requirements of accreditation agencies, the nursing education program (or its parent institution) and the site at which the clinical activities are to take place. These are more fully explored in Chapter 6, but a few aspects highly relevant to use of diverse sites are reviewed here.

Faculty members must ensure that state law, regulations, and rules related to faculty ratios, nature of faculty guidance, and student scope of practice are followed. Must the site be approved by the board of nursing? Is a specific contract required? Must the faculty member be present for clinical learning experiences for direct patient care to occur? Can preceptors be used in the setting being explored and in the manner planned? Can the instructor delegate guidance and evaluation of students' learning to an RN on staff at the agency if the instructor is not present but in the building? What if the instructor is not physically present?

Does the nursing education program have rules or policies related to these clinical placements? Is there a specific type of contract required? If faculty members must travel between sites, is travel reimbursement available? If the planned clinical learning activity will take place over more than the usual hours and day of a traditional clinical activity for that nursing education program (e.g., on parts of most days of the week depending on each student's rotation rather than all on 1 or 2 days over fixed hours), is this more time-intensive level of responsibility reflected in the faculty members' workload and compensation? Are there specific requirements of the education program's accreditation body (e.g., National League for Nursing Accrediting Commission, Commission on Collegiate Nursing Education) that affect the planned clinical learning activity?

What are the agency's rules and policies? Does the agency require a contract with the nursing education program? If so, who handles contracts with education programs? This a very important point for agencies that usually do not negotiate such contracts and where there is no clearly identified contact person. Some agencies that appear to be freestanding may actually be part of larger agencies. Where the agency is part of a larger entity (e.g., a hospital system, local government program, state health department, school district, or federal agency such as the Veterans Administration), it can be both difficult and time-consuming to get the contract signed by all relevant parties.

How are requests for clinical placements from multiple nursing education and other programs handled? This information is especially important when dealing with smaller agencies that may not have procedures in place to avoid conflicts when multiple programs (nursing and other health professionals) are seeking placements for the same time period.

What are the agency rules for student clearance (e.g., criminal background, child or elder abuse records, drug screening)? If screenings or background checks beyond the requirements of the nursing education program are required, who pays for them? Does the nursing education program need to document that students hold cardiopulmonary resuscitation or other certifications? What are the health requirements such as tuberculosis testing or immunizations? Are there specific Health Insurance Portability and Accountability Act (HIPAA) or client privacy statements that must be signed by each student? Does the agency need to keep a record of students for legal or regulatory purposes or to obtain future funding based on the value of student service to the organization? And which of these are also required of faculty members? Again, the policy of the larger organization of which the site where the students are placed is a part may predominate. In some cases the policy may require student orientation or check-off on items very peripheral or even irrelevant to the learning activity, but because students are at one of the entity's sites, the policy for the overall entity must be followed.

What is the required orientation? On the one hand, smaller and nontraditional sites (e.g., day care settings, church programs, food kitchens) and even some formal agencies that do not have large staffs (e.g., day treatment program for substance abusers, nursing home, assisted living facility) often do not require or have a formal orientation program. The faculty member will need to work with the staff to determine what preparation the students need to optimize their learning as well as to protect and provide the best care for the clients they will encounter. On the other hand, a larger institution (e.g., a major hospital system) may be the parent organization of smaller community-based programs, and students may need to complete the full agency orientation to be placed in even a small very peripheral program in the agency in addition to participating in a site-specific orientation. If these requirements become too onerous, expensive, or time-consuming, the value of clinical learning activities at these sites may be questioned by the nursing education program faculty and administration.

Preparation Requirements

Agency Preparation.   Details of the clinical learning activity (when will students be there, what their learning goals are) must be communicated with the staff. Settings that rarely host nursing students and those that often have nursing students can both have problems getting this information to the staff. Misunderstandings about student activities and objectives are common. Often student syllabi, clinical objectives, and guides to the clinical learning activity are provided to staff members who are not directly working with the students. A meeting with the staff and provision of multiple copies of these materials will facilitate communication.

Staff members and teachers need to identify a location for students to leave coats and other personal belongings in addition to a location for student conferences. Where these facilities are not available, alternatives will have to be identified.

Faculty Preparation.   Faculty members may need additional education, mentoring, and support as they implement clinical learning activities in some diverse settings. A highly skilled faculty member who is totally at ease teaching students to care for acutely ill clients in a critical-care unit may not have the knowledge and skills needed to care for those clients in their homes a week after discharge while they are still getting IV antibiotics. Like their students, faculty members may find that the fine points of adapting care to the home setting while respecting the family in their home and dealing with the virtual loss of the multiple support systems of the acute-care setting will be new to them.

Gaines, Jenkins, and Ashe (2005) reported on a program to teach faculty members about the Early and Periodic Screening, Diagnosis, and Treatment Program (EPSDTP), the use of the Denver II Developmental Screening Tool (DDST-2), and vision and hearing screening. Specific faculty members attended one or more programs to become certified in the tool or area. They then worked together to certify additional faculty members and the students who would be implementing the screenings. All nine participants received trainer certification from the state department of health for vision and hearing screening. Five faculty members traveled to Denver, Colorado, to receive certification as master instructors for the DDST. Two faculty members completed a 5-day program on THSteps (Texas's version of the EPSDT program) and were approved to provide the THSteps course.

Organization and structure of clinical teaching outside of acute care settings will often be new to a faculty member. Some logistical issues will need to be addressed. If the students are not all in the same setting, how will faculty members do their clinical teaching activities at multiple sites; how will students and teachers communicate with each other; how will clinical conferences occur; what clinical paperwork will be submitted to the faculty member, and when and how; and how and when will it be returned to students? A faculty mentor would facilitate the adjustment of faculty members new to the experience.

Regardless of the answers to these questions, faculty members who teach nursing students in diverse sites, perhaps at different sites at the same time, have more complex obligations than those working in a single site. For some sites, particularly those that are community-based or international, work beyond the days, times, or even weeks when traditional clinical learning activities occur may be needed to maintain partnerships. Small grant funding, for example from the local Area Health Education Consortium, can be used to pay faculty members for these additional responsibilities (Wink, 2003).

Student Preparation.   When students have clinical learning activities in sites that are different from those with which they are familiar, or where the learning opportunities are not immediately obvious to them, they often report that expectations are not always clear. In a study of factors that influence learning, Baillie (1993) found that prior experience at the site, the students' expectations and personal approach, and their relationship with their preceptors all were important to the quality of the experience. In addition, students reported that their preceptors' attitudes and knowledge, professional credibility, and skill as teachers had an impact on their learning. The specific placement, including perceived relevance of the placement to the course and student learning needs, the availability of relevant learning experiences, and practical aspects such as how far the placement is from the student's home all influenced learning (Baillie, 1993). Provision of specific objectives, learning activities, preparation expectations, activity guides, and written expectations will greatly facilitate learning and make the expectations clear, especially if the faculty member will not be present at the site at all times. See Table 15.1 for an example of site-specific preparation, objectives, activities, and written expectations for a community-based experience.

Orientation is based on agency, site, and student needs. Regardless of where each student will be, a global orientation to the course expectations with a review of skills used frequently in the experiences will get everyone started at a good pace. While each student will need orientation to the site where major clinical learning activities will take place, brief visits to each site used will help all members of the group put things in perspective when issues and challenges of specific sites are discussed in conferences among the clinical group members.

Student safety will also need to be addressed. This is an issue in all clinical activities but it is especially important in situations in which students may be in an unfamiliar area, making home visits, or going alone or in small groups to clinical

TABLE 15.1   Examples of Instructions to Students and Objectives for Specific Clinical Sites

For All Clinical Learning Activities

- Review objectives and activities as listed for each assignment and do assigned reading before arrival at the site.
- Creation of a summary sheet of key facts or bringing existing guides (e.g., immunization schedules or classification of hypertension in adults) is highly recommended.
- Be at the site at the time indicated by your instructor.
- Wear your uniform.
- Bring black pen, stethoscope, notebook, and pocket reference books as appropriate for the clinical learning activity.
- Work with the staff for an optimal learning experience.
- Have contact information for your instructor (beeper, cell phone number, etc.) with you at all times

Note: Your instructor may provide additional objectives or instructions for a specific site.

Physician's Office and Health Care Clinic: Adult

This clinical learning activity will take place in a physician's office or an adult health care clinic to which you will return throughout the semester. Your instructor will visit the site each day and be available via beeper or cell phone the remainder of the time. You may complete assessments, documentation, and teaching as described below. You may administer immunizations, but no other medications, under the direct observation of the RN identified by your instructor.

Course objectives met by this clinical learning activity include

- complete comprehensive health assessments of clients across the life span;
- identify relationships between health status of specific clients and pharmacological and other interventions;
- implement client-specific teaching plans based on assessment data;
- interpret laboratory findings in relation to client status;
- collaborate with the interdisciplinary health care team to plan and implement care.

Specific preparation before the clinical learning activity starts:

1. Read Chapters 12, 13, 29 in the course text.
2. Complete and submit to your instructor the immunization review packet in your course syllabus.

Bring the following items with you:

- Adult immunization schedule (http://www.cdc.gov/mmwr/PDF/wk/mm5345-Immunization.pdf)

(continues)

TABLE 15.1   Examples of Instructions to Students and Objectives for Specific Clinical Sites (Continued)

- Recommendations for cholesterol (total cholesterol, LDL, HDL, triglycerides) and blood pressure (http://www.clevelandclinicmeded.com/diseasemanagement/nephrology/hypertension/table1htn.htm)
- Recommendations for selected adult health screenings (p. 440 of text)
- Adult BMI chart (http://www.consumer.gov/weightloss/bmi.htm)
- List of common lab test normal values: hemoglobin, glucose, HGB A1C (look in the appendix of text)
- Form to use to record the drug names and dosages so that you can complete the follow-up assignment on drugs (you create this!)

Objectives

At the completion of this clinical learning activity, students will be able to do the following:

- Identify local demographics and social trends that are influencing the dynamics and structure of the contemporary adult/older family.
- Analyze the normative changes and non-normative events that challenge adults and older families
- Measure, record, and analyze vital signs, height, weight, BMI, and other assessment measurements.
- Conduct a focused health history with patients to determine chief concern, level of pain, nutritional needs, safety issues, medication regimen (names of drugs, dosages, frequency, any problems taking the medications reported by clients), and health promotion and immunization history.
- Record assessments on appropriate forms.
- Implement and document health education with individual clients and families.
- Explore information on the action, dosage range, nursing implications (including education needs), contraindications, cautions, and common side effects of selected medications.

Activities

During this clinical learning activity, students will work with staff members to accomplish the following:

- Follow agency policy for client intake for the visit, including completion of initial assessments and placement of clients and charts with appropriate provider.
- Review patient's chart for history, diagnoses, meds, lab test results.
- Follow patients through the physical exam to the end of the visit if provider and patient agree.
- Implement health teaching after review with the RN identified by your instructor.
- Administer immunizations under the direct observation and guidance of the RN identified by your instructor.

TABLE 15.1   (Continued)

Follow-up

At the completion of this clinical learning activity the students will perform the following actions:

- Discuss client interaction observations individually with the instructor or during clinical conference.
- Discuss client issues and needs identified during visits individually with the instructor or during clinical conference.
- Use a drug handbook to look up three medications taken by clients met at the office or clinic and record
  - name of the drug (brand and generic),
  - usual indications (reason) for the drug being given,
  - why this client is getting the drug,
  - side effects of the drug,
  - usual dosage.
- Submit the medication findings at the end of your journal for the week.
- Complete one SOAP note based on a client encounter during this clinical learning activity and submit it with your journal for the week.
- Complete a nursing care plan for one client problem identified during this clinical learning activity and submit it with your journal for the week.

Source: Adapted with permission from the University of Central Florida School of Nursing.

sites. Teachers must provide explicit guidelines for student safety during learning activities and document them in the course syllabus. Safety guidelines for home visits and going alone or in small groups to clinical sites should address communication with faculty, agency and client, including emergency contact information, need for clear travel directions and a reliable vehicle, and appropriate dress and behavior while in a client's home or at an agency or facility without an instructor present. The students must also be prepared for action needed if in a dangerous situation, be it at an agency, out in the community, or at a client's home (Reed & Wuyscik, 1998).

To facilitate student preparation and safety in community-based settings, the University of Alberta developed a four-prong program. The first component is a detailed student checklist including activities that were part of preparation for the visit (personal preparation, agency preparation, and vehicle preparation) and the implementation of the visit (environmental surveillance and personal response to situations). The other three components were a set of four small-group learning discussions on topics such as examining risky situations and responses, a Web-based module, and a problem-based learning tutorial (Skillen, Olson & Gilbert, 2003).

SUMMARY

Nursing care occurs anywhere there are clients who need the services of a professional nurse, and nursing students can learn to provide care wherever they have contact with clients. Traditionally, much of clinical nursing education has occurred in acute-care settings because of long-held assumptions about how nurses must be prepared to practice. However, decreasing length of inpatient stays, high patient acuity, economic pressures to provide care in outpatient and community settings, and increasing competition with other educational programs for the same clinical sites have limited clinical learning opportunities located in traditional acute-care settings. Using diverse sites for clinical learning activities would prepare nursing students for the challenges of contemporary nursing practice as clients, health needs, care locations, and approaches to care evolve.

This chapter discussed options for planning and providing clinical learning opportunities for undergraduate and graduate nursing students in a wide variety of clinical sites. Examples of clinical learning opportunities in three categories were presented. The first category included patient care areas that are not used regularly as clinical learning sites (e.g., the operating room, outpatient clinics, nursing homes) despite the rich learning opportunities for students in these settings. The second category included sites where provision of health care is not the prime focus of the site or agency, such as schools, camps, and apartment complexes. The third category is the growing use of international clinical learning opportunities.

Practical aspects of clinical placements in diverse sites also were discussed. Two main areas of concern are the need to meet regulatory and accreditation requirements and the need for adequate preparation of the agency, faculty, and students. Examples of methods and tools used for preparation of agency staff members, faculty members making the transition from traditional acute care sites, and nursing students were provided.

REFERENCES

AORN. (2006). *The value of clinical learning activities in the perioperative setting in undergraduate nursing curricula* [position statement]. Retrieved June 1, 2006, from http://www.aorn .org/about/positions/pdf/POS-Value%20of%20Clinical%20Learning.pdf

Arrington, D. T. (1997). Retirement communities as creative clinical opportunities. *N & HC: Perspectives on Community, 18,* 82–85.

Baillie, L. (1993). Factors affecting student nurses' learning in community placements: A phenomenological study. *Journal of Advanced Nursing, 18,* 1043–1053.

Button, L., Green, B., Tengnah, C., Johansson, I., & Baker, C. (2005). The impact of international placements on nurses' personal and professional lives: Literature review. *Journal of Advanced Nursing, 50,* 315–324.

Caffrey, R. A., Neander, W., Markle, D., & Stewart, B. (2005). Improving the cultural competence of nursing students: Results of integrating cultural content in the curriculum and an international immersion experience. *Journal of Nursing Education, 44*, 234–240.

Chen, S., Melcher, P., Witucki, J., & McKibben, M. (2002). Nursing home use for clinical rotations. Taking a second look. *Nursing and Health Sciences, 3*, 131–137.

Crigger, N., & Holcomb, L. (in press). Practical strategies for providing culturally sensitive, ethical care in developing nations. *Journal of Transcultural Nursing.*

DeLashmutt, M. B., & Rankin, E. A. (2005). A different kind of clinical experience: Poverty up close and personal. *Nurse Educator, 30*, 143–149.

Duffy, M. E., Farmer, S., Ravert, P., & Huittinen, L. (2004). International community health networking project: Two year follow-up of graduates. *International Nursing Review, 52*, 24–31.

Frank, B., Adams, M., Edelstein, J., Speakman, E., & Shelton, M. (2005). Community-based nursing education of prelicensure students: Settings and supervision. *Nursing Education Perspectives, 26*, 283–286.

Gaines, C., Jenkins, S., & Ashe, W. (2005). Educational innovations. Empowering nursing faculty and students for community service. *Journal of Nursing Education, 44*, 522–525.

Goetz, M. A., & Nissen, H. (2005). Educational innovations. Building skills in pediatric nursing: Using a child care center as a learning laboratory. *Journal of Nursing Education, 44*, 277–279.

Grant, E., & McKenna, L. (2003). International clinical placements for undergraduate students. *Journal of Clinical Nursing, 12*, 529–535.

Hayes, A. (2005). A mental health nursing clinical experience with hospice patients. *Nurse Educator, 30*, 85–88.

Hitt, S. F., & Overbay, J. D. (1997). Educational innovations. Maximizing the possibilities: Pediatric nursing education in non-traditional settings. *Journal of Nursing Education, 36*, 339–341.

Kavanagh, K. H. (1998). Summers of no return: Transforming care through a nursing field school. *Journal of Nursing Education, 37*, 71–79.

Kiehl, E., & Wink, D. M. (2000). Nursing students as change agents and problem solvers in the community. *Nursing and Health Care Perspectives, 21*, 293–297.

Kurtz, S., & Eichelberger, L. W. (1999). Developing a perioperative nursing elective. *AORN Journal, 70*, 879–886.

Ligeikis-Clayton, C., & Denman, J. Z. (2005). Clinical issues. Service-learning across the curriculum. *Nurse Educator, 30*, 191–192.

Matteson, P. (Ed.). (1995). *Teaching nursing in the neighborhoods. The Northeastern University model.* New York: Springer Publishing.

Matteson, P. (Ed.). (2000). *Community-based nursing education. The experiences of eight schools of nursing.* New York: Springer Publishing.

Mitchell, L., Stevens, M., Goodman, J., & Brown, M. (2002). Establishing a collaborative relationship with a college of nursing. *AORN Journal, 76*, 842–848.

Oneha, M. F., Magnussen, L., & Feletti, G. (1998). Ensuring quality nursing education in community-based settings. *Nurse Educator, 23*, 26–31.

Reed, F. C., & Wuyscik, M. A. (1998). Teach what? Reflections on the transition from hospital teaching to teaching in the community. *Nurse Educator, 23*, 11–13.

Resick, L. K., Taylor, C. A., Carroll, T. L., D'Antonio, J. A., & de Chesnay, M. (1997). Establishing a nurse-managed wellness clinic in a predominantly older African American inner-city high rise: An advanced practice nursing project. *Nursing Administration Quarterly, 21*, 47–54.

Riner, M. E., & Becklenberg, A. (2001). Partnering with a sister city organization for an international service-learning experience. *Journal of Transcultural Nursing, 12*, 234–240.

Ross, C. A. (1998). Preparing American and Nicaraguan nurses to practice home health nursing in a transcultural experience. *Home Health Care Management and Practice, 11*, 65–69.

Ryan, S. A., D'Aoust, R. F., Groth, S., McGee, K., & Small, A. L. (1997). A faculty on the move into the community. *Nursing and Health Care Perspectives, 18*, 139–141, 149.

Sigsby, L. (2004). Perioperative clinical learning experiences. *AORN Journal, 80*, 476, 479, 481–490.

Sigsby, L., & Yarandi, H. (2004). A knowledge comparison of nursing students in perioperative versus other rotations. *AORN Journal, 80*, 699–707.

Skillen, D., Olson, J., & Gilbert, J. (2003). Promoting personal safety in community health: Four educational strategies. *Nurse Educator, 28*, 89–94.

Tagliareni, M. E., & Speakman, E. (2003). Community-based curricula at the ADN level: A service-learning model. In M. Oermann & K. Heinrich (Eds.), *Annual review of nursing education* (Vol. 1, pp. 27–41). New York: Springer Publishing.

Tanner, C. (2006). The next transformation: Clinical education. *Journal of Nursing Education, 45*, 99–100.

Taylor, C. A., Resick, L., D'Antonio, J. A., & Carroll, T. L. (1997). The advanced practice nurse role in implementing and evaluating two nurse-managed wellness clinics: Lessons learned about structure, process, and outcomes. *Advanced Practice Nursing Quarterly, 3*, 36–45.

Thompson, K., Boore, J., & Deeny, P. (2000). A comparison of an international experience for nursing students in developed and developing countries. *International Journal of Nursing Studies, 37*, 481–492.

Toften, K., & Fonnesbeck, B. (2002). Camp communities: Valuable clinical options for BSN students. *Journal of Nursing Education, 41*, 83–85

Wink, D. (2003). Community-based curricula at BSN and graduate levels. In M. Oermann & K. Heinrich (Eds.), *Annual review of nursing education* (Vol. 1, pp. 3–25). New York: Springer Publishing.

Wolf, K. A., Goldfader, R., & Lehan, C. (1997). Women speak: Healing the wounds of homelessness through writing. *N & HC: Perspectives on Community, 18*, 74–78.

World Health Organization. (2002). *Promoting rational use of medicines: Care components.* Geneva: World Health Organization.

Zotti, M., Brown, P., & Stotts, R. (1996). Community-based nursing versus community health nursing: What does it all mean? *Nursing Outlook, 44*, 211–217.

Chapter 16

Clinical Evaluation and Grading

In clinical evaluation the teacher assesses the extent of students' learning and quality of performance in clinical practice. Evaluation is an essential component of clinical teaching. Through the evaluation process the teacher confirms that the competencies have been developed and the student can progress to other learning outcomes or assesses continued learning needs, requiring further instruction by the teacher or more practice by the student. This chapter highlights important principles of clinical evaluation and guides readers in how to evaluate and grade students in the practice setting.

WHAT IS CLINICAL EVALUATION?

Clinical evaluation is a process by which judgments are made about the learner's performance in clinical practice. Performance may be assessed in a practice setting where students are caring for patients, families, and communities; through a simulation; or in a learning or skills laboratory. Clinical evaluation involves observing the student's performance and arriving at judgments about the quality of that performance based on the competencies to be evaluated. There are two phases in clinical evaluation: (1) observing students' performance and collecting other data about student learning in the course and (2) based on those observations and data, determining if the student achieved the clinical competencies. Clinical evaluation is subjective because it involves making a judgment about performance based on the teacher's observations and other data.

This chapter was adapted from chapters 12, 13, and 16 in Oermann, M. H., & Gaberson, K. B. (2006). *Evaluation and testing in nursing education* (2nd ed.). New York: Springer. Adapted by permission of Springer Publishing Company, Inc., New York.

Clinical Evaluation Versus Grading

Clinical evaluation is not the same as grading. In evaluation the teacher observes performance and collects other types of data about student learning, then compares this information to a set of standards to arrive at a judgment. A quantitative symbol or grade may be applied to reflect the evaluation data and judgments made about the student's performance. The clinical grade, such as pass–fail or A through F, is the symbol that represents the evaluation data and teacher's judgments. Clinical performance may be evaluated and not graded, for example, when the teacher gives feedback to the learner and does not incorporate those observations with the final rating of performance. Grades, however, should never be assigned without sufficient observations and data about the student's performance and learning in the course.

Norm- and Criterion-Referenced Clinical Evaluation

Clinical evaluation may be norm- or criterion-referenced. In *norm-referenced evaluation*, the student's clinical performance is compared to other students in the clinical group, indicating that the performance is better than, worse than, or equivalent to the other students in the comparison group. A clinical evaluation form in which students' performance is rated as above-average, average, or below-average would be an example of a norm-referenced interpretation.

In contrast, *criterion-referenced clinical evaluation* involves comparing the student's clinical performance to predetermined criteria, not to the performance of other students in the group. Criterion-referenced evaluation indicates that the student has achieved the clinical competencies or met the course outcomes regardless of how other students performed in the course.

Formative and Summative Clinical Evaluation

Clinical evaluation may be formative or summative. *Formative evaluation* in clinical practice provides feedback to learners about their progress in developing the clinical competencies. The purposes of formative evaluation or feedback are to enable students to develop their clinical knowledge and skills and identify areas in which further learning is needed. With this type of evaluation, instruction is provided to move students forward in their learning. Formative evaluation, therefore, is diagnostic and is not graded (Nitko, 2004). For example, the clinical teacher or preceptor might observe a student perform wound care and give feedback on changes to make with the technique. The goal of this evaluation is to improve subsequent performance, not to grade how well the student carried out the procedure.

Summative clinical evaluation, however, is designed for determining clinical grades because it summarizes competencies the student has developed in clinical practice. Summative evaluation is done at the end of the clinical practicum or another point in time to assess the extent to which learners have achieved the clinical competencies. Summative evaluation is not diagnostic; it summarizes the performance of students often using rating scales or another type of clinical evaluation form. For much of clinical practice in a nursing program, summative evaluation comes too late for students to have an opportunity to improve performance.

Any protocol for clinical evaluation should include extensive formative evaluation and periodic summative evaluation. Formative evaluation is essential to provide feedback to improve performance while practice experiences are still available.

FAIRNESS IN THE EVALUATION OF NURSING STUDENTS

Considering that clinical evaluation is subjective, the goal is to establish a *fair* evaluation system. Fairness requires that the teacher

- identify own values, beliefs, and biases that may influence the evaluation process;

- base the clinical evaluation process on the clinical competencies and course outcomes;

- develop a supportive clinical learning environment.

Identify Own Values

Teachers need to be aware of their personal values, beliefs, and biases that may influence evaluating students' performance. These can affect both the data collected about students and the judgments made. In addition, students have their own set of values and attitudes that influence their self-assessment of performance and their responses to the teacher's feedback. The teacher may need to intervene to guide students in more self-awareness of their own values and the effect they are having on learning.

Base Clinical Evaluation on the Clinical Competencies or Course Outcomes

Clinical evaluation should be based on the competencies, clinical objectives, or course outcomes to be met in clinical practice—these guide the evaluation process. Without these, neither teacher nor student has any basis for what to evaluate in clinical practice. For example, if the competencies relate to developing communication skills, then the learning activities, whether in the patient care setting or laboratory, should assist students in learning how to communicate. The teacher's observations and subsequent evaluation should focus on communication behaviors, not on other competencies unrelated to the learning activities.

Develop a Supportive Learning Environment

The teacher needs to develop a supportive learning environment in which students view the teacher as someone who will facilitate their learning and development of clinical competencies. Students need to be comfortable asking faculty and staff questions and seeking their guidance rather than avoiding them in the clinical setting. A supportive environment is critical for effective evaluation because students need to recognize that the teacher's feedback is intended to help them improve performance. A supportive learning environment includes developing trust and respect between teacher and students (Chan, 2003).

IMPORTANCE OF FEEDBACK

For clinical evaluation to be effective, the teacher should provide continuous feedback to students about their performance and how they can improve it. This feedback may be verbal, by describing observations of performance and explaining what to do differently, or visual, by demonstrating correct performance. Feedback should be accompanied by further instruction from the teacher or by directing the student to other resources for learning. The ultimate goal is for students to judge their own performance and locate resources for their learning.

There are five principles for providing feedback to students as part of the clinical evaluation process. First, the feedback should be precise and specific. General information about performance, such as "You need to work on your assessment" or "You need more practice" does not indicate what behaviors need improvement nor how to develop them. Instead of using general statements, the teacher should indicate the specific areas of knowledge that are lacking and competencies that need more development.

Second, for procedures and any technical skill, the teacher should provide both verbal and visual feedback: The teacher should explain first, either orally or in writing, where the errors were made in performance and then demonstrate the correct procedure or skill. Then the student should practice the skill with the teacher guiding performance. By allowing immediate practice, with the teacher available to correct problems, students can more easily *use* the feedback to further develop their skills.

Third, feedback about performance should be given to students at the time of learning or immediately following it. The longer the period of time between performance and feedback from the teacher, the less effective is the feedback. As time progresses, neither student nor teacher can remember specific areas of clinical practice to be improved. This principle holds true whether the performance relates to critical thinking and decision making, a procedure or technical skill, or an attitude or value expressed by the student. With the hectic pace of many clinical settings and number of students in a clinical group, the teacher needs to develop a strategy for giving focused and immediate feedback to students during the clinical day and following up with further discussion as needed. Recording short notes on paper, in personal digital assistants (PDAs), or on flow sheets for later discussion with individual students helps the teacher remember important points about performance.

Fourth, students need different amounts of feedback and positive reinforcement. In beginning practice and with clinical situations that are new to learners, most students will need frequent feedback. As students progress through the nursing program, they should be assessing their own performance and seeking guidance less frequently from the teacher. Some students need more feedback and direction from the teacher than others. As with many aspects of education, one approach does not fit all students.

One final principle is that feedback should be diagnostic: After identifying areas in which further learning is needed, the teacher's responsibility is to guide students so they can improve performance. The process is cyclical—the teacher observes and evaluates performance, gives students feedback about that performance, and then guides their learning and practice so they can become more competent.

CLINICAL EVALUATION STRATEGIES

There are many evaluation strategies that can be used for assessing clinical performance and other learning outcomes in clinical practice. Some evaluation strategies are appropriate for use by faculty or preceptors who are on-site with students and can observe their performance; other evaluation methods assess students' knowledge, cognitive skills, and other competencies but do not involve direct observation of performance. Some methods, such as journals, are best for formative evaluation while others are useful for either formative or summative evaluation.

There are several factors to consider when selecting clinical evaluation strategies to use in a course. First, the evaluation methods should provide information about student performance of the clinical competencies associated with the course. With the evaluation strategies, the teacher collects data on performance to judge if students are developing the clinical competencies or have achieved them by the end of the course. For many outcomes of a course, there are different strategies that can be used, thereby providing flexibility in choosing methods for evaluation. In planning the evaluation for a clinical course, the teacher should review the competencies to be developed and decide on evaluation strategies for assessing them, recognizing that most methods provide information on more than one competency or course outcome.

Second, the teacher should select evaluation strategies that are realistic considering the number of students to be evaluated, available practice or simulation activities, and constraints such as the teacher's or preceptor's time. Planning for an evaluation method that depends on patients with specific health problems or particular clinical situations may not be realistic considering the types of experiences with actual or simulated patients available to students. Some strategies are not appropriate because of the number of students who would need to use them within the time frame of the course. Others may be too costly or require resources not available in the nursing education program or health care setting.

Third, in the process of deciding how to evaluate students' clinical performance, the teacher should identify if the strategies will be used to provide feedback to learners (formative) or for grading (summative). Students should know this ahead of time.

Fourth, before finalizing the protocol for evaluating clinical performance in a course, the teacher should review the purpose and number required of each assignment completed by students in clinical practice. What are the purposes of these assignments, and how many are needed to demonstrate competency? For example, in some clinical courses students complete an excessive number of written assignments. How many assignments, regardless of whether they are for formative or summative purposes, are needed to meet the outcomes of the course? Students benefit from continuous feedback from the teacher, not from repetitive assignments that contribute little to their development of clinical knowledge and skills. Instead of daily or weekly care plans or other assignments, which may not even be consistent with current practice, once students develop the competencies, they can progress to other more relevant learning activities.

Fifth, in deciding how to evaluate clinical performance, the teacher should consider his or her own time for completing the evaluation and providing feedback to students. Instead of requiring a series of written assignments in a clinical course, the same outcomes might be met through discussions with students, cases analyzed by students in clinical conferences, group writing activities, and other methods requiring less faculty time and accomplishing the same purposes. Considering the demands on nursing faculty, it is important to consider personal time when planning how to evaluate students' performance in clinical practice (Oermann, 2004).

Observation

The main strategy for evaluating clinical performance is observing students in clinical practice, simulation and learning laboratories, and other settings. Although observation is widely used, there are threats to its validity and reliability. Observations of students may be influenced by the teacher's values, attitudes, and biases. In any performance assessment the teacher needs to make a series of observations before arriving at judgments about performance.

In observing performance, the teacher can direct attention to many aspects of that performance. For example, while observing a student administer an intravenous medication, the teacher can focus on the technique used for its administration or how the student interacts with the patient. Another teacher observing this same student may focus on other aspects of the performance. The same practice situation, therefore, may yield different observations. Because of these differences, the teacher should focus the observation on the clinical competencies being evaluated; these guide what the teacher looks for in observing student performance. It is also important to discuss observations with students, obtain their perceptions of behavior, and be willing to modify personal inferences when new data are presented. Otherwise the teacher may arrive at incorrect judgments about student performance.

Every observation of a student is only a sampling of the learner's performance during a clinical activity. An observation of the same student at another point in time may reveal a different level of performance. Therefore, the teacher should observe performance more than once before arriving at conclusions about the student's competencies.

Faculty members need a strategy to help them remember their observations of students and the context in which the performance occurred. There are several ways of recording observations of students in clinical settings, simulation and learning laboratories, and other settings: anecdotal notes, checklists, and rating scales.

Anecdotal Notes.   Anecdotal notes are narrative descriptions of observations made of students. Walsh and Seldomridge (2005) emphasized the importance of writing complete and accurate anecdotal notes to substantiate the clinical grade. Some faculty members include only a description of their observations of students, and then, after a series of observations, they review the pattern of performance and draw conclusions about it. Other faculty members record their observations and include a judgment about how well the student performed (Case & Oermann, 2004). Anecdotal notes should be recorded as close to the time of the observation as possible; otherwise it is difficult to remember what was observed and the context, for example, patient and clinical situation, of that observation. In the clinical setting, notes can be handwritten on flow sheets, on other forms, or as narratives. They also can be recorded in PDAs.

Anecdotal notes should be shared with students as frequently as possible; otherwise they are not effective for feedback. The teacher should discuss observations with students and be willing to incorporate the students' own judgments about performance. Anecdotal notes are also useful in conferences with students, for example, at midterm and end of term, as a way of reviewing a pattern of performance over time. When there are sufficient observations about performance, the notes can serve as documentation for ratings on the clinical evaluation tool.

Checklists.   A checklist is a list of specific behaviors or activities to be observed with a place for marking whether or not they were present during the performance (Nitko, 2004). It often lists the steps to be followed in performing a procedure or demonstrating a skill. Checklists allow faculty to observe procedures and behaviors performed by students, but they also provide a way for students to assess their own performance. For common procedures and skills, teachers can often find checklists already prepared that can be used for evaluation, and some nursing textbooks have accompanying skills checklists.

Rating Scales.   Rating scales, also referred to as clinical evaluation tools or instruments, provide a means of recording judgments about observed performance of students in clinical practice. A rating scale has two parts: (1) a list of competencies, behaviors, or outcomes the student is to demonstrate in clinical practice and (2) a scale for rating their performance of them.

Rating scales are most useful for summative evaluation of performance; after observing students over a period of time, the teacher can rate their performance according to the scale provided with the instrument. Table 16.1 provides guidelines for using rating scales for clinical evaluation in nursing.

There are many types of rating scales for evaluating clinical performance. Many schools of nursing use pass–fail or satisfactory–unsatisfactory scales. Rating scales also can be multidimensional such as A, B, C, D, E; 1, 2, 3, 4, 5; exceptional, above-average, average, and below-average; and always, usually, frequently, sometimes, and never. Nitko (2004) suggested that multidimensional scales include a short description with the letters, numbers, and labels to improve objectivity

TABLE 16.1   Guidelines for Using Rating Scales for Clinical Evaluation

1. Be alert to the possible influence of your own values, attitudes, beliefs, and biases in observing performance and drawing conclusions about it.
2. Use the clinical outcomes, competencies, or behaviors to focus your observations. Give students feedback on other observations made about their performance.
3. Collect sufficient data on students' performance before drawing conclusions about it.
4. Observe the student more than one time before rating performance. Rating scales when used for clinical evaluation should represent a *pattern* of the students' performance over a period of time.
5. If possible, observe students' performance in different clinical situations either in the patient care or simulated setting. When not possible, develop additional strategies for evaluation so performance is evaluated with different methods and at different points in time.
6. Do not rely on first impressions; they may not be accurate.
7. Always discuss observations with students, obtain their perceptions of performance, and be willing to modify your own judgments and ratings when new data are presented.
8. Review the available clinical learning activities and opportunities in the simulation and learning laboratories. Are they providing sufficient data for completing the rating scale? If not, new learning activities may need to be developed or the behaviors on the tool may need to be modified to be more realistic considering the clinical teaching circumstances.
9. Avoid using rating scales as the only source of data about a student's performance—use multiple evaluation methods for clinical practice.
10. Rate each outcome, competency, or behavior individually based on the observations made of performance and conclusions drawn. If you have insufficient information about achievement of a particular competency, do not rate it—leave it blank.
11. Do not rate all students high, low, or in the middle; similarly, do not let your general impression of the student or personal biases influence the ratings.
12. If the rating form is ineffective for judging student performance, then revise and reevaluate it. Consider these questions: Does use of the form yield data that can be used to make valid decisions about students' competence? Does it yield reliable, stable data? Is it easy to use? Is it realistic for the types of learning activities students complete and available in clinical settings?

Source: Reprinted from Oermann, M. H., & Gaberson, K. B. (2006). *Evaluation and testing in nursing education* (2nd ed.). New York: Springer, p. 222, by permission of Springer Publishing Company, Inc., New York.

and consistency. For example, for the competency "Collects relevant data from patients," descriptors for the exceptional level (or A or 1) might be "differentiates relevant from irrelevant data," "analyzes multiple sources of data," "establishes comprehensive database," and "identifies data needed for evaluating all possible nursing diagnoses and patient problems." Examples of a satisfactory–unsatisfactory and a multidimensional tool for clinical evaluation are presented as Figures 16.1 and 16.2.

Simulations

Simulations are another strategy for clinical evaluation. With simulations students can demonstrate procedures, conduct assessments, analyze clinical scenarios and make decisions about problems and actions to take, carry out care, and evaluate the effects of their decisions. Each of these outcomes can be evaluated for feedback to students or for summative grading.

Simulations can be developed with models and manikins for evaluating skills and procedures. With human patient simulators (HPSs), faculty can identify outcomes and clinical competencies to be evaluated, present various clinical events and situations on the simulator for students to analyze and take action, and evaluate student decision making and performance in these scenarios.

Many nursing education programs have set up simulation laboratories with HPSs, clinically equipped examination rooms, manikins and models for skill practice and assessment, areas for simulated patients, and a wide range of multimedia that facilitate performance evaluations. The rooms can be equipped with two-way mirrors, video cameras, microphones, and other media for observing and rating performance by faculty and others. Videoconferencing technology can be used to conduct clinical evaluations of students in settings at a distance from the nursing education program, effectively replacing on-site performance evaluations by faculty.

One type of simulation for clinical evaluation uses standardized patients. Standardized patients are individuals who have been trained to accurately portray the role of a patient with a specific diagnosis or condition. With simulations using standardized patients, students can be evaluated on a history and physical examination, related skills and procedures, and communication techniques, among other outcomes. Standardized patients are effective for evaluation because the actors are trained to recreate the same patient condition and clinical situation each time they are with a student, providing for consistency in the performance evaluation. When standardized patients are used for formative evaluation, they provide feedback to the students, an important aid to their learning.

Perioperative Nursing
Clinical Performance Evaluation

Name _____ Date _____

OBJECTIVE	S	U
1. Applies principles of aseptic technique		

A. Demonstrates proper technique in hand antisepsis, gowning, gloving
   B. Prepares and maintains a sterile field
   C. Recognizes and reports breaks in aseptic technique		

2. Plans and implements nursing care consistent with *AORN Standards and Recommended Practices for Perioperative Nursing*		

A. Collects physiological and psychosocial assessment data preoperatively
   B. Identifies nursing diagnoses for the perioperative period based on assessment data
   C. Develops a plan of care based on identified nursing diagnoses and assessment data
   D. Provides nursing care according to the plan of care
   E. Evaluates the effectiveness of nursing care provided
   F. Accurately documents perioperative nursing care		

3. Provides a safe environment for the patient		

A. Assesses known allergies and previous anesthetic incidents
   B. Adheres to safety and infection control policies and procedures
   C. Prevents patient injury due to positioning, extraneous objects, or chemical, physical, or electrical hazards		

4. Prepares patient and family for discharge to home		

A. Assesses patient's and family's teaching needs
   B. Teaches patient and family using appropriate strategies based on assessed needs
   C. Evaluates the effectiveness of patient and family teaching
   D. Identifies needs for home care referral		

5. Protects the patient's rights during the perioperative period		
A. Provides privacy throughout the perioperative period B. Identifies and respects the patient's cultural and spiritual beliefs		

FIGURE 16.1   Sample clinical evaluation tool using satisfactory–unsatisfactory scale. (*Source:* Adapted from Oermann, M. H., & Gaberson, K. B. (2006). *Evaluation and testing in nursing education* (2nd ed.). New York: Springer, p. 324; by permission of Springer Publishing Company, Inc., New York.)

Clinical Evaluation Form

Total Raw Score: _____   Faculty Name: _____

Student Name: _____   Letter Grade: _____

Mean Score: _____   Agency: _____

	4	3	2	1	na
Uses a theoretical framework in care of individuals, families, and groups in the community					
A. Applies concepts and theories in the practice of community health nursing					
B. Examines multicultural concepts of care as they apply to the community					
C. Analyzes family theory as a basis for care of clients in a community setting					
D. Examines relationships of family members within a community setting					
E. Examines the community as a client through ongoing assessment					
F. Evaluates health care delivery systems within a community setting					
Uses the nursing process for care of individuals, families, and groups in the community and the community as client					
A. Adapts assessment skills in the collection of data from individuals, families, and groups in a community setting					

FIGURE 16.2   Sample clinical evaluation tool using multidimensional scale. (*Source:* Tool developed by Judith M. Fouladbakhsh, MSN, APRN, BC, AHN-C, CHTP, and Effie Hanchett, PhD, RN. Adapted by permission of J. Fouladbakhsh and E. Hanchett, 2005. Reprinted from Oermann, M. H., & Gaberson, K. B. (2006). *Evaluation and testing in nursing education* (2nd ed.). New York: Springer, pp. 354–355; by permission of Springer Publishing Company, Inc., New York.)

Clinical Evaluation Form (Continued)

	4	3	2	1	na
B. Uses relevant resources in the collection of data in the community					
*C. Analyzes client and community data					
D. Develops nursing diagnoses for individuals, families, and groups within the community and the community as a client					
E. Develops measurable outcome criteria and plan of action					
F. Uses outcome criteria for evaluation plans and effectiveness of interventions					
*G. Assumes accountability for own practice in the community					
H. Uses research findings and standards for community-based care					
*I. Accepts differences among clients and communities					
Is responsible for identifying and meeting own learning needs					
*A. Evaluates own development as a professional					
*B. Meets own learning needs in community practice					

FIGURE 16.2   (Continued)

Clinical Evaluation Form (Continued)

	4	3	2	1	na
Collaborates with others in providing community care					
A. Interacts effectively with clients and others in the community					
B. Uses community resources effectively					

*Critical behaviors must be rated at least at 2.0 to pass clinical practicum.

4 = Consistently excels in performance of behavior; independent

3 = Is competent in performance; independent

2 = Performs behavior safely; needs assistance

1 = Unable to perform behavior; requires guidance all the time

na = Not applicable

Faculty and Student Narrative

Faculty Comments:

Signature:_____ Date _____

Student Comments:

Signature:_____ Date _____

FIGURE 16.2   Sample clinical evaluation tool using multidimensional scale. (Continued)

Objective Structured Clinical Examination

An Objective Structured Clinical Examination (OSCE) provides a means of evaluating performance in a simulation laboratory rather than the clinical setting. In an OCSE students rotate through a series of stations (Newble & Reed, 2004). At each station they complete an activity or perform a task, which is then evaluated. Some stations assess the student's ability to take a patient's history, perform a physical examination, and implement other interventions while being observed by the teacher or an examiner. The student's performance can then be rated using a rating scale or checklist. At other stations, students might be tested on their knowledge and cognitive skills—they might be asked to analyze data, select interventions and treatments, and manage the patient's condition. Most often OSCEs are used for summative clinical evaluation; however, Alinier (2003) describes how they can be used formatively to enhance skill acquisition among nursing students.

Written Assignments

Written assignments accompanying the clinical experience are effective strategies for evaluating students' problem solving, critical thinking, and higher-level learning; understanding of content relevant to clinical practice; and ability to express ideas in writing. Many types of written assignments for clinical courses are described in Chapter 13: concept map, concept analysis paper, short written assignments, nursing care plan, case method and study, evidence-based practice papers, teaching plan, journal, group writing, and portfolio. These assignments can be included as part of the clinical evaluation. Some will be evaluated formatively, such as journals, while others can be graded. The teacher should first specify the outcomes to be evaluated with written assignments and then decide what assignments would best assess if those outcomes were met.

Portfolios

A portfolio is a collection of projects and materials developed by the student that documents achievement of the competencies and outcomes of the clinical course. Portfolios are valuable for clinical evaluation because students provide evidence in their portfolios to confirm their clinical competencies and document new learning and skills acquired in a course. The portfolio can include evidence of student learning for a series of clinical experiences or over the duration of a clinical course. Portfolios can be evaluated and graded by faculty based on predetermined criteria. They can also be used for students' self-assessment of their progress in meeting personal and professional goals.

Nitko (2004) identified two types of portfolios: best-work, and growth and learning progress. Best-work portfolios provide evidence that the student has demonstrated certain competencies and achievements in clinical practice; these are appropriate for summative clinical evaluation. Growth and learning-progress portfolios are designed for monitoring students' progress and self-reflection of learning outcomes at several points in time. These contain products and work of the students in process for faculty to review and provide feedback (Nitko, 2004).

For clinical evaluation, these purposes can be combined. The portfolio can be developed initially for growth and learning, with products and entries reviewed periodically by the faculty for formative evaluation, and then as a best-work portfolio with completed products providing evidence of clinical competencies. The best-work portfolio can then be graded. Because portfolios are time-consuming to develop, they should be used for determining if students met the outcomes and passed the clinical course and should be graded rather than prepared only for self-reflection.

The contents of the portfolio depend on the outcomes of the clinical course and competencies to be achieved. Many types of materials and documentation can be included in a portfolio. For example, students can include short papers that they completed in the course, a term paper, reports of group work, reports and analyses of observations made in the clinical setting, self-reflections of clinical experiences, and other products they developed in their clinical practice. The key is for students to choose materials that demonstrate their learning and development of clinical competencies. By assessing the portfolio, faculty should be able to determine if students met the outcomes of the course.

Conferences

There are many types of conferences appropriate for clinical evaluation depending on the outcomes to be met. Preclinical conferences take place prior to beginning a clinical learning activity and allow students to clarify their understanding of patient problems, interventions, and other aspects of clinical practice. In those conferences, faculty can assess students' knowledge and provide feedback to them. Postclinical conferences, held at the end of a clinical learning activity or a predetermined point in time during the clinical practicum, provide an opportunity for faculty to evaluate students' ability to use concepts and theories in patient care, plan care, assess the effectiveness of interventions, problem solve and think critically, collaborate with peers, and achieve other outcomes depending on the focus of the discussion.

Most conferences are evaluated for formative purposes, with the teacher giving feedback to students as a group or to the individual who led the group discussion.

When conferences are evaluated as a portion of the clinical or course grade, the teacher should have specific criteria to guide the evaluation and should use a scoring rubric.

Group Projects

Most of the clinical evaluation strategies presented in this chapter focus on individual student performance. Group projects can also be assessed as part of the clinical evaluation in a course. Some group work is short term—only for the time it takes to develop a product such as a teaching plan or group presentation. Other groups may be formed for the purpose of cooperative learning with students working in small groups or teams in clinical practice over a longer period of time. With any of these group formats, both the products developed by the group and ability of students to work cooperatively can be assessed.

There are different approaches for grading group projects. The same grade can be given to every student in the group, that is, a group grade, although this approach does not take into consideration individual student effort and contribution to the group product. Another approach is for students to indicate in the finished product the parts they contributed to, providing a way of assigning individual student grades with or without a group grade. Students can also provide an assessment of how much they contributed to the group project, which can then be integrated into their grade. Alternately, students can prepare both a group and an individual product. Nitko (2004) emphasized that rubrics should be used for evaluating group projects and should be geared specifically to the project.

To assess students' participation and collaboration in the group, the rubric also needs to reflect those goals of group work. With small groups, the teacher can observe and rate individual student cooperation and contributions to the group. However, this approach is often difficult because the teacher is not a member of the group, and the group dynamics change when the teacher is present. As another approach, students can evaluate the participation and cooperation of their peers. These peer evaluations can be used for the students' own development and shared among peers but not with the faculty, or can be incorporated by the teacher in the grade for the group project. Students can also be asked to assess their own participation in the group.

Self-Evaluation

Self-evaluation is the ability of students to assess their own clinical performance and competencies and identify both strengths and areas for improvement. Faculty should hold planned conferences with each student to review self-evaluations with the students. In these conferences faculty can give specific feedback on clinical performance, elicit the student's own perceptions of competencies, identify strengths and areas for learning from the teacher's and student's perspectives, and plan learning activities for improving performance.

GRADING CLINICAL PRACTICE

Grading systems for clinical practice are often two-dimensional, such as pass–fail, satisfactory–unsatisfactory, and met–did not meet the clinical objectives. Some programs add a third category, honors, to acknowledge performance that exceeds the level required. Other grading systems are multidimensional, for example, using letter grades, A through F; integers, 1 through 5; and percentages. With any of these grading systems, it is not always easy to summarize the multiple types of evaluation data collected about the student's performance into a symbol representing a grade. Even in a pass–fail system it may be difficult to arrive at a judgment as to pass or fail based on the evaluation data and the circumstances associated with the student's clinical and simulated practice.

Categories for grading clinical practice such as pass–fail and satisfactory–unsatisfactory have some advantages over a multidimensional system although there are disadvantages as well. Pass–fail places greater emphasis on giving feedback to the learner because only two categories of performance need to be determined. With a pass–fail grading system faculty members may be more inclined to provide continual feedback to learners because they do not have to ultimately differentiate performance according to four or five levels of proficiency such as with a letter system. Performance that exceeds the requirements and expectations, though, is not reflected in the grade for clinical practice unless a third category is included: honors pass–fail. Alfaro-LeFevre (2004) reported from her survey of 79 nursing programs, which were randomly selected, that a pass–fail grading system was used in 59 (75%) of the programs. Fifteen (15%) programs assigned letter grades for the clinical practicum.

A pass–fail system requires only two types of judgment about clinical performance: Do the evaluation data indicate that the student has demonstrated satisfactory performance of the competencies to indicate a pass? Or do the data suggest that the performance of those competencies is not at a satisfactory level? Arriving at a judgment as to pass or fail is often easier for the teacher than using the same evaluation information for deciding on multiple levels of performance. A letter system for grading clinical practice, however, acknowledges the different levels of clinical proficiency students may have demonstrated in their clinical practice.

Regardless of the grading system for clinical practice, there are two criteria to be met: (1) the evaluation strategies for collecting data about student performance should reflect the clinical competencies and outcomes for which a grade will be assigned and (2) students must understand how their clinical practice will be evaluated and graded. In planning the course the teacher needs to decide which of the evaluation strategies should be incorporated in the clinical grade. Some of these strategies are for summative evaluation, thereby providing a source of information for including in the clinical grade. Other strategies, though, are used in clinical practice for feedback only and are not incorporated in the grade.

Methods for Assigning the Clinical Grade

Once the grading system is determined, there are varied ways of using it to arrive at the clinical grade. The grade can be assigned based on the competencies or outcomes achieved by the student. To use this method the faculty should consider designating some of the competencies or outcomes as critical for achievement in the course. For example, an A might be assigned if all of the clinical competencies or outcomes were met; a B might be assigned if all of the competencies designated by faculty as critical behaviors and at least half of the others were met.

For pass–fail grading faculty can indicate that all of the competencies or outcomes must be met to pass the course or can designate critical behaviors required for passing the course. In both methods, the clinical evaluation strategies provide the data for determining if the student's performance reflects achievement of the competencies. These evaluation strategies may or may not be graded separately as part of the course grade.

Another way of arriving at the clinical grade is to base it on the evaluation strategies. In this system the clinical evaluation strategies become the source of data for the grade. For example,

Paper on analysis of clinical practice issue	10%
Analysis of clinical cases	5%
Conference presentation	10%
Community resource paper	10%
Portfolio	25%
Rating scale (of performance)	40%

Observation of performance, and the rating on the clinical evaluation tool, is only a portion of the clinical grade. An advantage of this approach is that it incorporates into the grade the summative evaluation methods completed by students. If pass–fail is used for grading clinical practice, the grade might be computed as follows:

Paper on analysis of clinical practice issue	10%
Analysis of clinical cases	5%
Conference presentation	10%
Community resource paper	10%
Portfolio	25%
Clinical examination, simulations	40%
Rating scale (of performance)	Pass required

This discussion of grading clinical practice suggests a variety of mechanisms that are appropriate. The teacher must make it clear to students and others how the evaluation and grading will be carried out in clinical practice, through simulations, and in other settings.

Failing Clinical Practice

Teachers will be faced with determining when students have not met the outcomes of the clinical practicum, that is, have not demonstrated the competencies to pass the clinical course. There are principles that should be followed in evaluating and grading clinical practice, which are critical if a student fails a clinical course or has the potential for failing it. Following are some of these principles; further information is available in Oermann and Gaberson (2006).

- The evaluation strategies used in a clinical course; how each will be graded, if at all; and how the clinical grade will be assigned should be in writing and communicated to students.
- If failing clinical practice means failing the nursing course, this consequence should be stated clearly in the course syllabus and policies. By stating it in the syllabus, which all students receive, students have it in writing before clinical learning activities begin.
- Students should sign any written clinical evaluation documents—anecdotal notes, rating forms (of clinical practicum, clinical examinations, and performance in simulations), narrative comments about the student's performance, and summaries of conferences in which performance was discussed. Their signatures do not mean they agree with the ratings or comments, only that they have read them. Students should have an opportunity to write in their own comments.

- Students need continuous feedback on their clinical performance. Observations made by the teacher, the preceptor, and others and evaluation data from other sources should be shared with the student. Together they should discuss the data. Students may have different perceptions of their performance and in some cases may provide new information that influences the teacher's judgment about clinical competencies.

- When the teacher or preceptor identifies performance problems and clinical deficiencies that may affect passing the course, conferences should be held with the student to discuss these areas of concern and to develop a plan for remediation. It is critical that these conferences focus on problems in performance combined with specific learning activities for addressing them. One of the goals of the conference is to develop a plan with learning activities for the student to correct deficiencies and develop competencies further. The plan should include a statement that one "good" or "poor" performance will not constitute a pass or fail clinical grade and that sustained improvement is needed (Graveley & Stanley, 1993). The plan should also indicate that completing the remedial learning activities does not guarantee that the student will pass the course, and that the student must demonstrate satisfactory performance of the competencies by the end of the course.

- Students with the potential of failing clinical practice may have other problems affecting their performance. Faculty should refer students to counseling and other support services and not attempt to provide these resources themselves.

- As the clinical course progresses, the teacher should give feedback to the student about performance and continue to guide learning. It is important to document the observations made, other types of evaluation data collected, and the learning activities completed by the student. The documentation should be shared routinely with students, discussions about performance should be summarized, and students should sign these summaries to confirm that they read them.

- There should be a policy in the nursing program about actions to be taken if the student is unsafe in clinical practice. If the practice is safe even though the student is not meeting the outcomes, the student is allowed to continue in the clinical practicum (Graveley & Stanley, 1993) because the clinical competencies and outcomes are identified for achievement at the *end* of the course not during it. If the student demonstrates performance that is potentially unsafe, however, the teacher can remove the student from the clinical setting following the policy and procedures of the nursing program. Specific learning activities outside of the clinical setting need to be offered for students to develop the knowledge and skills they lack; practice with simulators is valuable in these situations. A learning plan should be prepared and implemented as described earlier.

- In all instances the teacher must follow the policies of the nursing program. If the student fails the clinical course, the student must be notified of the failure and its consequences as indicated in these policies. The teacher must know the policies and follow them with all students (Boley & Whitney, 2003).

SUMMARY

In clinical evaluation the teacher makes a judgment about the student's performance in clinical practice. The teacher's observations should focus on the competencies to be developed in the clinical course or the outcomes to be met. The competencies or outcomes provide the framework for learning in clinical practice and the basis for evaluating performance. Teachers also need to examine their own values, beliefs, and biases because these may affect their evaluation of students. Effective clinical evaluation requires a supportive learning environment and continuous feedback from the teacher.

Many clinical evaluation strategies are available for use in a nursing course. The teacher should choose evaluation methods that provide information on student performance of the clinical competencies. The teacher also decides if the evaluation strategy is intended for formative or summative evaluation.

The predominant method for clinical evaluation is observing the performance of students in clinical practice and recording the observations in anecdotal notes, on checklists, and on rating scales. With simulations students can demonstrate procedures, conduct assessments, analyze clinical scenarios, and make decisions about problems and actions to take. Each of these outcomes can be evaluated for feedback to students or for summative grading.

There are many types of written assignments useful for clinical evaluation depending on the outcomes to be assessed. Written assignments can be developed as a learning activity and not evaluated, reviewed by the teacher for formative evaluation, or graded.

A portfolio is a collection of materials that the student developed in clinical practice over a period of time. With portfolios, students provide evidence to confirm their clinical competencies and document the learning that occurred in the clinical setting.

Other clinical evaluation methods are conference, group project, and self-evaluation. The evaluation methods presented in this chapter provide the teacher with a wealth of strategies from which to choose in evaluating students' clinical performance.

Important guidelines for grading clinical practice and working with students who have the potential for failing a clinical course were discussed in the chapter. These guidelines give direction to teachers in establishing sound grading practices and following them when working with students in clinical practice.

REFERENCES

Alfaro-LeFevre, R. (2004). Should clinical courses get a letter grade? *The Critical Thinking Indicator, 1*(1), 1–5. Retrieved from http://www.alfaroteachsmart.com/clinicalgrade newsletter.pdf

Alinier, G. (2003). Nursing students' and lecturers' perspectives of objective structured clinical examination incorporating simulation. *Nurse Education Today, 23,* 419–426.

Boley, P., & Whitney, K. (2003). Grade disputes: Considerations for nursing faculty. *Journal of Nursing Education, 42,* 198–203.

Case, B., & Oermann, M. H. (2004). Clinical teaching and evaluation. In L. Caputi & L. Engelmann (Eds.), *Teaching nursing: The art and science* (pp. 126–177). Glen Ellyn, IL: College of DuPage Press.

Chan, D. S. K. (2003). Validation of the Clinical Learning Environment Inventory. *Western Journal of Nursing Research, 25,* 519–532.

Graveley, E. A., & Stanley, M. (1993). A clinical failure: What the courts tell us. *Journal of Nursing Education, 32,* 135–137.

Newble, D., & Reed, M. (2004). *Developing and running an Objective Structured Clinical Examination (OSCE).* Retrieved January 25, 2005, from http://www.shef.ac.uk/~dme/oscehandbook.doc

Nitko, A. J. (2004). *Educational assessment of students* (4th ed.). Upper Saddle River, NJ: Prentice Hall.

Oermann, M. H. (2004). Reflections on undergraduate nursing education: A look to the future. *International Journal of Nursing Education Scholarship, 1*(1), 1–15. Retrieved from http://www.bepress.com/ijnes/vol1/iss1/art5

Oermann, M. H., & Gaberson, K. B. (2006). *Evaluation and testing in nursing education* (2nd ed.). New York: Springer Publishing.

Walsh, C. M., & Seldomridge, L. A. (2005). Clinical grades: Upward bound. *Journal of Nursing Education, 44,* 162–168.

Index